CORE DIET
FOR KIDS
SECOND EDITION

Stephen J. Gislason, M.D.

The most important book ever written for the understanding and
management of children's food related problems

VOLUME 3 OF THE NUTRITIONAL MEDICINE SERIES

 PerSona Audiovisual Productions

Copyright ©1989 Stephen J. Gislason & Environmed Research Inc.

First Edition 1988
Second Edition 1989

Canadian Cataloguing in Publication Data

    Gislason, Stephen J., 1943 – The core diet for kids
        (Nutritional medicine series / Stephen J.Gislason; 3)
        Includes bibliographical references
        ISBN 0-9694145-0-1

        1. Food allergy in children – Diet therapy. 2. Diet
        therapy for children. 3. Children – Nutrition. I.
        Title. II. Series:Gislason, Stephen J., 1943 –
        Nutritional Medicine Series;3.
        RJ386.5.G581989   618.92'00654   C89-091518-0

Nutritional Medicine Series
Volume 1. Manual for Professionals
      2. The Core Diet
      3. The Core Diet for Kids
      4. Core Diet Cooking
      5. Nutritional Programming
      6. Headache Therapy
      7. Neuropsychiatry and Diet Revision Therapy

Published by:
    PerSona Audiovisual Productions
    #1-3661 West 4th Ave. Vancouver, B.C.
    V6R 1P2 (604) 731-9168

Cover Photo of: Soren Gislason
Printers: Hignell Printing
Typesetting: PerSona Audiovisual Prod.
Illustrations: Pamela Fajardo, BSc. & Magee
Engineering & Graphic Design

ACKNOWLEDGMENTS

My patients have inspired this work. The plight of suffering children who are misunderstood and even blamed for their illnesses have touched me deeply. I am especially grateful to all the mothers who are tireless in their search for solutions to their children's problems. Some mothers (more than fathers) are heroic in their selfless efforts. They have contributed much of the information and insight written in this book. I am grateful to Drs. Justin Parr and David Stinson for their insightful teachings and the view of medicine as the synthesis of compassion and scientific rigor.

The insights and research of many physicians and scientists are also represented in this book. I have based my understanding of food allergy mechanisms on the work of many physicians and scientists that I do not know personally - the research reports of W. A. Hemmings first alerted me to the passage of intact proteins through the intestinal wall and the distribution of these protein to body tissues, especially the brain. I then discovered the pioneers in the clinical observation of food allergy patterns - Drs. Walter Alvarez, Philip Gottlieb, M. Brent Campbell, Fredrick Speer, Theron Randolph, A.H. Rowe, H.J. Rinkel, W. Rea, Marshall Mandel, and Doris Rapp were especially helpful early on in confirming the general validity of my clinical observations. The work and writings of Drs. J.W. Garrard, R.Reinhardt, R.R.A. Coombs, P. McLaughlin, John Beinstock, A.S. McNeish, D.J. Atherton, Jonathan Brostroff, William Knicker, R. Pagnelli, Joseph Egger, Iris Bell, L. Businco, Claudio Carini, J.A. Bellanti, J.F. Soothill, Georges Halpern, W. Allen Walker, their associates, and many others were especially helpful in my search for explanations for the wide range of food allergic patterns in my patients.

The friendship and intellectual support of Dr. Mort Low and Barbee Low has been invaluable - I may never have persisted in the difficult pursuit of unpopular, but correct, solutions to health problems without their encouragement. Claire Alston was generous with her help and support in the intial stages of writing "Molecular Programming", a precursor to the Core Diet work. Chuck Bates and Carla Van Dam have successfully incorporated diet revision therapy into the practice of clinical psychology. Chuck's writing and enthusiastic support of my work is gratefully acknowledged. Dr. Julianne Conry has been a supportive colleague and co-researcher. Dr. Tanya Wulff recently joined our team of insighful enthusiasts and has been marvellously supportive. Linda Gomez contributed much to family support in our children's study, and Liz Harris taught us about family compliance in the difficult task of diet revision. Barb Keating has brought her personal and teacher's insights into the problem of allergic disease to educational practice and has established a model for the effective and compassionate management of sensitive children at school. Ula Timmermanns has returned to contribute her experience, editing and formatting, helping again to bring this text to fruition. Pamela Fajardo contributed illustrations and cover design to the second addition and has added her boost of skills and enthusiasm to the Nutritional Medicine project. Thank you all.

Preface to Revised Edition 2

Children suffer needlessly. One common source of their distress is improper food and drink. There are many causes of food-related illness, but the solution to all food problems is the same - effective diet revision.

The Core Diet program is a successful therapeutic approach to the management of a wide range of food-related illnesses. The program is presented in this book along with explanatory essays, with the hope that more parents and their children will have access to this safe and effective solution to health problems. The text has been written as simply as possible without compromising the accuracy of the instructions nor the informative value of the explanatory texts.

The theory behind the Core Diet incorporates scientific concepts which you should find interesting. The professional reader should benefit from the clear description of a successful clinical method of resolving common illnesses, and may consult companion tests for more information. Core Diet recommendations are based on empirical evidence and sound biological information - not speculation, preference, or opinion.

The Core Diet program is human software. The program can and should be modified by parents, according to the special needs of each child. It is a flexible program of permanent diet revision for sustained good health. As you reconstruct your child's food supply from a hypoallergenic clearing diet, you decide every day if your child's response to food is okay or not okay. If it is not okay, you modify food choices until your child feels better, and then proceed with further food introductions.

The first rule of medical therapy is to *do no harm*. Diet Revision Therapy is motivated by kindness and love.

Section 1 of this book reviews the important reasons why so many children are sick in our modern, affluent societies and why their food supply is a major factor in creating their disturbances and illnesses. We review the specific indications for diet revision therapy.

Section 2 is a complete instruction set. The Core Diet method is described in detail. This instruction set should allow an intelligent, well-motivated parent to undertake successful diet revision for his or her child. The critical phase of the Core Diet is a clearing program, followed by a careful, well-tested food reintroduction sequence. Common experiences on this path are described, along with basic instructions for problem-solving.

The Core Diet often works uneventfully if the instructions are carefully followed. Many parents will succeed in solving their child's problems. Some children are more complicated than others and difficulties may persist. There are too many problems to cover all possibilities in this text. My role, as the supervising physician, is to provide help in troubleshooting, symptom interpretation, problem-solving, behavioral management, and supportive counselling. Without knowledgeable professional supervision, you may encounter some difficulties which you cannot readily solve. Professional supervision is highly recommended.

Section 3 provides more information about food, its interaction with your child's body, and the mechanisms of illness. The essays in Section 3 are intended as introductions to the science supporting the Core Diet method. The section begins with a mini-course on feeding infants and children. Chapters 6 and 7 are brief, pertinent reviews of feeding policies and basic nutrition. Chapter 8 describes the gastrointestinal tract (GIT) and its digestive functions. Chapter 9 reviews the subject of food additives. Chapters 10 through 12 will help you understand the complicated subject of food allergy. Chapters 13 and 14 introduce you to the effect of food on emotions, behavior, and learning ability. Examples of Core Diets, and their nutritional analyses, are included in the appendices. My guess is that if you read Section 3 material several times during your experiences with diet revision, it will all eventually make sense to you. You may soon want more complete information. Further discussion of these topics may be found in "The Core Diet", a parallel program for adults; "Core Diet Cooking", a meal-planning and recipe book; and "Nutritional Programming", a more technical treatise for professional readers and experienced parents.

May you bring greater health, peace, and happiness to the lives of your children.

Stephen J. Gislason, MD

Vancouver, British Columbia
Canada, August 1989

Contents

THE CORE DIET FOR KIDS

Section 1

**Introduction to Food Related Illnesses
and Diet Revision Therapy**

**The Children Who Will Benefit from
the Core Diet**

Glossary of Terms

CCHO	Complex Carbohydrates
CFP	Carbohydrate,Fat,Protein prop.
CHOL	Cholesterol
CHO	Carbohydrate
DRT	Diet Revision Therapy
ENF	Elemental Nutrient Formula
EFA	Essential Fatty Acid
FA	Fatty Acid
FAL	Food Allergy
GIT	Gastrointestinal Tract
IDI	Ill Defined Illness
IMD	Immune Mediated Disease
MP	Molecular Programming
NDP	Nutrient Disproportion
NP	Nutritional Programming
NUMED	Nutritional Medicine
RDA	Recommended Daily Allowance

Chapter 1

INTRODUCTION TO THE CORE DIET

This book is about helping sick and disturbed children get better by changing their food supply. It is also about the nature of food problems.

Jane Brody, a well-known journalist and author of excellent nutrition books[1,2] recently wrote in the New York Times:

> "Researchers studying the often-surprising effects of nutrition on immunity report that dietary manipulation can be a promising new tool to foster recovery or prevent disease in millions of people."

Brody's interest is focused on biochemical and immunological discoveries. She mentions the fatty acid, EPA, in its immune modulating or anti-inflammatory role and other interesting nutritional details. While I share her interest and enthusiam for the "nice possibilities" of biochemical intervention in disease, I am also aware of the hidden, sinister aspects of our experience. Our biggest, most menacing problems are in our food supply and our polluted damaged environment. I spend my days treating individual patients, both children and adults, who are sick and suffering, often from a mysterious illness.

Children are among our most vulnerable citizens since they breathe in polluted air and consume a wide variety of food materials that no previous generation of human beings has ever experienced. Often their food makes them ill and we need to be deeply concerned.

Parents want explanations, better diagnosis and treatment from physicians, and action from politicians to remedy environmental problems. They want relief from chemical contamination of food. They want protection for their children who are also getting ill in mysterious and complicated ways.

1.0.1 Why Are Children Ill?

We continue to discover abject ignorance about food-caused illness among professionals who really should know better. The problem is not just ignorance of basic biology, ecology, biochemistry, and toxicology, but also a belligerent denial of the sickness and suffering of fellow human beings. This ignorance and denial is all the more unacceptable as planet-wide biological emergencies become obvious. We must not deny the growing evidence of atmospheric crises, climate changes, and widespead pollution of the food chain.

In groups, we often make terrible mistakes and rely on people in authority who lack the competence, leadership, and ability to get us out of trouble. We have made a few broad assumptions about the nature and cause of disease which are probably wrong. We will either change these assumptions or perish from them.

We assume that psychosomatic illness is common, and explains most human problems we do not understand. And we are wrong.

We assume that "stress" is the cause of most illness and define stress in social and emotional terms. And we are wrong.

We assume that unexplained physical illness is "in the mind", has psychosocial causes, or is mysterious and unsolvable. And we are wrong.

We assume that mental illness has either psychosocial causes or is mysterious. We deny that mental illness has biological causes and that the most important biological causes are in the food supply, the air, and water. We deny that chemical pollution causes mental illness. We deny that noise, bad lighting, crowding, and smelly, polluted air causes mental illness. And we are wrong.

Moreover, we assume that we can pollute and destroy and natural environments without harm to ourselves. Or, in the best case, if we recognize that deterioration of the natural environment, we assume that it really does not make our children sick right now and we have a lot of time to fix it. And we are wrong.

We assume that physicians really know what is wrong with us and that drugs are the answer to all illness. We assume that medical technology is up-to-date and appropriate to the problems we are having today. And we are wrong.

What else can we think?

We can realize that we create problems as we solve others. That we need to change almost everything that we think and do. Those of us who care for and love children who become ill and dysfunctional need to change our own local habits and methods. We start with recognizing and solving the problems in our food supply.

The biological perspective in medicine, as it is now taught and practised, may be limited to specific details of organ function and ignore the large issues of our behavior, habitat, and maladaptation to planet Earth.

Alternative healing systems are even more negligent in solving biological problems and settle for fantasies and wishful thinking. Unfortunately much nutritional "healing" advice comes more from fantasy that effective biology.

Environmental quality is the major biological concern. It is normal for a biologist to think in terms of populations, food supply, seasons, weather, and social-behaviours, and to do field studies which reveal patterns of adaptation to specific environments.

The biologist sees every living creature connected to and interacting with his/her environment. Anyone who has worked with animals or fish in closed environments knows how critical environmental conditions and diet are in determining both the behavior and the physical status of the residents. When a fish in an aquarium displays psychotic behaviour, you do not call a fish psychiatrist; you check the oxygen concentration, temperature, and pH of the water. You have to clean the tank and change the fish diet.

A steady flow of molecules from the environment enters the body of each individual, through the air breathed and the food and liquids ingested. A whole-systems approach to medicine studies this molecular stream. We assume that body-input determines not only health and disease in the long-term, but also the moment to moment functional capacity of the individual. Our destiny, individually and collectively, can swerve dramatically with changes in this molecular stream.

We all live in and interact with home and work environments which determine our biological fate. In industrialized countries, the micro-environment of each person is controlled by human constructions and is generally polluted by toxic substances (the extent of which is seldom measured) which are little understood. As environmental problems multiply new ill-defined illnesses will increase.

Biological systems tend to absorb adverse changes for a time, then collapse precipitously. We can expect therefore and explosive increase in food-related and environmental illness in the next decade or two. The food supply will carry the greatest burden of environmental problems. The immediate toxicity of air pollution, increased UV radiation, surface warming, acid rain and chemical contamination of the food supply are the most conspicuous environmental problems. Virus evolution is tied to global changes and will likely produce a series of novel endemic diseases - AIDS is a model of the next round of infectious illness.

Food and ingested liquids are selected by socioeconomic and cultural factors more than biological factors. Food selection is part of more complex behavioral patterns often determined by television advertising and the intense availability of junk and fast foods. Children are exposed to relentless advertising efforts which easily convince them to seek biologically bad food and establish maladaptive eating patterns. Common abnormal eating behaviours include cravings, compulsions, binge-eating, continued excessive food intake with obesity, food addictions, aversions, and anorexia.

The quality and composition of air, food, and water changes continuously. The illusion of food continuity that the supermarket presents to us conceals the changes in the growth, contamination, storage, spoiling, transportation, and merchandising of food products. The air we breathe is in constant flux and may vary from tolerable to toxic. To understand environmental reactivity, we must deal with changes, variability, and inconsistencies, and seek adaptive flexible responses to changing circumstances.

1.0.2 Diet Revision as Therapy

Since disease may arise from dysfunctional food-body interactions, diet revision is a remarkably successful and safe method of treatment. Food produces illness and dysfunction in a variety of ways.

No medical specialty has assumed the clinical responsibility of applying knowledge of environmental principles, ecology, or toxicology. Allergists intend to understand the medical problems of the environment, but often limit their knowledge and practice to a few selected environmental problems, like hay fever or asthma. Too often, medical investigations, including X-rays and blood tests, are inadequate to diagnosis complex food-related illness patterns in children. Many parents have been told that the lab tests are normal "... so there is nothing wrong". If your physician cannot make a clinical diagnosis or appreciate the complexities of your child's metabolic machinery and its many opportunities to malfunction, you may search in vain for an effective solution to your child's health problems.

Diet revision therapy to the rescue: an attempt to correct food supply problems would often be more helpful than extensive (expensive) medical investigation and futile drug treatments.

The Core Diet is a program of diet reconstruction that works in clinical practice and may be useful to many people who seek solutions to their health problems. The Core Diet, for example, can usually solve the problem of migraine headaches - a disease that causes great suffering and incurs considerable expense. If a drug were discovered which would "cure" migraine, it would be announced triumphantly in headlines and TV specials. Diet revision is safe, cost-effective, and brings you many free-bonus benefits. It only costs the effort to make changes in habits and expectations.

The first goal of Diet Revision Therapy (DRT) is curative - to resolve illness and dysfunction by reconstructing a healthier diet, free of problems that commonly cause dysfunction and disease. The second goal is preventive - to avoid dysfunction and disease by maintaining a low risk diet.

The Core Diet is
* a successful therapeutic method of diet revision
* helpful in resolving dysfunction and disease
* a flexible program of designing a new safe food supply
* a program of permanent change in food selection habits

The Core Diet is not
* a fixed or rigid program of food selection
* a weight loss program
* a temporary solution to short-lived problems

The original design of the Core Diet was based on the managment of food allergy - a complex of problems in children that are poorly understood, seldom diagnosed, and seldom managed properly. The best reason for beginning diet revision is to help a child feel and function better. Intelligent parents with the help of well-informed physicians should be capable of resolving many complex illness patterns in children which otherwise cause much suffering and life-long dysfunction. Discussion of patterns of food allergy and other food-related illness follow in this and next chapters.

1.0.3 Food Allergy

Many diseases may arise from dysfunctional food-body interactions. Our main concern is food allergy, a collection of serious disease patterns caused by immune-system responses to food. Allergy is immune-mediated dysfunction and disease. The allergic process may be the most common cause of disease in the Western world. Food allergy probably afflicts everyone. This is a heretical conviction that still meets opposition. Food allergy often co-exists with digestive and absorption disturbances, metabolic, and biochemical problems. Since food allergy is the underlying cause of many common illnesses suffered by our children, we shall understand that an attempt to correct faulty food (body-input) problems by diet revision is a safe and effective therapy.

Food allergy disturbances are surprising in intensity and variety. Symptom patterns can be sorted into the body systems expressing the greatest disturbance, or we can sort problems in other ways - according to the underlying food chemistry, metabolic mistake, or immune mechanism involved. Symptoms tend to occur in pattern clusters and in sequences which tell us something about the defensive mechanisms in our body. We often suffer from the well-intentioned defense responses of the intestinal tract and the immune system.

There are many different patterns of allergic disease. Food allergy is not one entity or pattern. Food allergy is a name used to describe a host of immune responses to food materials in the digestive tract, blood, and tissue spaces. Some physicians talk about allergy only in terms of "atopic" patterns of allergy - eczema, hay fever, asthma, hives, and swelling reactions. The range of food allergic illness extends well beyond atopic illnesses. An oversimplified, but convenient description of allergic patterns separates immediate hypersensitivity allergy from the less obvious and more complex "delayed" patterns of illness. Immediate food reactions, like lip/mouth swelling or vomiting, are obviously connected to food intake, but the food connection to a delayed symptom, like headache or disturbed behavior, may not be apparent at all. The patterns of immediate hypersensitivity are distinct from the delayed responses to food ingestion, but synergism seems to exist.

A common presentation of delayed pattern food allergy in my practice is a child who suffers many recurrent symptoms over several years, often beginning in infancy. Nose congestion (rhinitis) and flushing (red cheeks and ears) are the two most common symptoms. Dark circles around the eyes are known as "allergic shiners" and conspicuously mark the children with food allergy. An astute observer can make the diagnosis of food allergy from across the room. Often tonsils, adenoids, and the neck lymph nodes are enlarged; these immune-system organs are stimulated by food allergens ingested every day, and enlarge to defend the body against the perceived "enemies" in food. The throat is often sore, with increased mucus production. Many children snort, cough, clear their throat frequently, and snore at night. The middle ear is continuous with the nose and throat and intermittently fills with fluid. Regularly, middle-ear fluid feeds local bacteria and an ear infection develops with severe pain and loss of hearing. Many food-allergic children suffer permanent hearing loss. We refer to the complex of ear-nose-throat food allergy symptoms as CURS - Chronic Upper Respiratory Syndrome.

Often respiratory symptoms are associated with headaches, stomach aches, leg pains, rashes, hives, eczema, irritablity, sleep disturbances, nightmares, bed wetting, and many other disturbances. Restless or hyperactive behavior may be linked to temper tantrums, moodiness, crying, fighting, and defiance and low self esteem.

Allergy to things in the air is often confused with food allergy. Symptom patterns may be similar, but the mechanisms are different. Sneezing, nose congestion, eye irritation may come from both airborne and food allergens at the same time, or at different times during the year. It is better to think of food allergy as a separate problem which might co-exist with, for example, hay fever.

The presentation of food allergy is often confused with infections - bacterial and viral - and the diagnosis may be "colds" or "flu". The child may be frequently ill with non-specific symptoms. Antibiotics and cough and decongestion syrups are often prescribed. Food allergy is best diagnosed from the history of illness. The best clue to the diagnosis is the presence of many symptoms in many different parts of the body, over months to years. Food allergy often begins in infancy with colic, vomiting, diarrhea, skin rashes, and disturbed behavior. The patterns of illness evolve over the ensuing years. The disappearance of infant symptoms suggests that the child has "outgrown" food allergy, but often the problem has simply shifted from acute, obvious expressions to hidden, delayed symptoms. In making the diagnosis of food allergy, we look for typical signs of the disease - red cheeks and ears, blue circles around the eyes, nose stuffiness, enlarged tonsils and neck lymph nodes, and a variety of skin problems.

Skin tests often do not reveal the food allergy. Even if some skin tests are positive, these tests do not predict the response to foods eaten.

Further description of patterns of illness in Chapter 2 and several discussions in Section 3 will give you a better understanding of the complexities of food allergy.

The 14 most common symptoms in children with food allergy are:

Nose congestion	*Diarrhea or constipation*
Nose bleeds	*Itching, skin rashes, bumps*
Cough	*Fatigue*
Sore throat	*Leg pains*
Middle ear "infection"	*Moodiness, hyperactivity*
Headache	*Sleep disturbances*
Abdominal pain	*Difficulty concentrating*

If your child has 3 or more of these common symptoms on a regular or recurrent basis, they have delayed pattern food allergy until proven otherwise. If they have 3 or more of the following physical signs you can be even more certain of the food allergy diagnosis. (Skin tests cannot make the diagnosis of food allergy.)

The 10 most common physical signs of food allergy are:

Allergic shiners	*Edema (water retention)*
Flushing, face and ears	*Distended abdomen*
Throat inflammation	*Abdominal tenderness*
Enlarged neck glands	*Skin rashes, bumps, sores*
Nose lining swelling	*Eczema*

Allergy expresses itself as inflammation in body tissues, targeted by immune cells activated by food allergens. In medical descriptions, the suffix "itis" means inflammation. Thus, "rhinitis" means nose inflammation, "arthritis" means joint inflammation and so on. A simple rule of thumb is that any disease description ending in "itis" could be caused by food allergy. The description of patterns of food allergic illness are continued in Chapter 2.

Diet revision therapies must then be concerned with reducing or eliminating food allergy before any other motive for food selection come into play. The Core Diet has emerged from a systematic study of patients with food allergy. The plan works because it has been the best food choices for the best outcome for the most children. It is, in other words, a critical path of diet revision with the highest probability of success through the maze of possible food choices. The job of the parent with or without help for your physician and dietician is to determine which of the foods recommended on the Core Diet are safe and well-tolerated by each child. We are all different and the Core Diet must be tailored to custom-fit each child.

1.0.4 Social Implications of Diet Revision

One mother who successfully treated her son with the Core Diet program wrote about the politics and implications of her experience[3]:

"Three years ago... I began an Odyssey, consulting doctors and psychologists in search of explanations for my son's unpredictable and aggressive behavior. As a low income single parent my search has been prolonged by the inclination of professionals to consider psychosocial causes, rather than biological causes for my son's difficulties...as an infant (he had) colic, projectile vomiting and diarrhea...when he turned two...his usual sunny disposition was clouded by angry outbursts.. he would heave platefuls of food on the floor and overturn the kitchen table...by age three no behavioral management techniques I had learned were effective...

My son's future is brighter now due to a radical change in his diet...The change in my son has been positive and dramatic. His face is no longer pallid with flushed cheeks and ears. He doesn't breathe thru his mouth, his nose is clear, and he no longer has dark circles under puffy eyes. Other complaints such as leg pains, nausea, headache, diarrhea, fatigue and irritability are at bay. His attention deficit, mild hyperactivity, and mood-swings with anti-social aggressive behavior are under control. My son is adjusting well to the change in his diet. He prefers not to eat the food that give him, in his own words, "difficult feelings"".

1.0.5 Stress or Allergy?

Our environment changes continuously and we are required to adapt continuously. When the change is too great or too sudden, a failure of adaptation occurs, with malfunctioning of mind/body as a consequence. Any interaction between individual and environment which produces symptoms (is maladaptive) can be called "stress". Any event, agent or component of the environment which causes a maladaptive response is called a "stressor". Our children live in a perpetual state of adaptatation - growing, learning, succeeding, failing, suffering illness and injury. They live in a perpetual state of stress. Wrong food ingestion is likely to be the most common body stress that modern children suffer. If food input is neither predictable, nor controllable, major body stress occurs with all its negative consequences. You can think about this as you present all the packaged, bottled, canned foods, treats, and snacks to your children. If you were to become the child's body input manager, concerned about matching the flow of materials into your child's delicate biological machinery, how would you feel about the haphazard mix of raw materials, presented as the child's food and drink? What would you tell your supervisors when you were unable to produce reliable, high-quality products - good behavior, successful learning, disease prevention, happy, and healthy children?

The biological meaning of the word "stress" is often lost in popular usage. Emotional responses are not stressful, nor are emotions symptoms of stress. Hard work is not always stressful. The most stressful events are those changes in our environment and food which automatic control systems in us can neither control nor predict. Events which cause unstable changes in our body function require our adaptive responses. If our responses work, the instability is reduced and no stress occurs. If the responses do not work, then body systems, seeking balance, become confused, and maladaptive body-states and behaviors appear.

Hans Selye was the father of the stress concept. As a young scientist, he set out to learn more about how animals and people get sick. Intuitively, he took a whole-systems approach. The early ideas of "stress" were based on observations of physical changes in animals exposed to injury, prolonged pain, or to challenges with toxins and allergens. It is curious to review how the original idea of stress has been exaggerated in popular usage to describe all manner of relatively innocuous circumstances. Stress has become a mythical dragon, beyond any biological definition. A patient will describe "stress" when he has to work overtime, or when she has relatives visiting. All manner of emotional experiences and trivial discomforts are now called "stress".

Selye made important observations about allergic disease. In his 1956 book "The Stress of Life",[4] he described injecting rats with egg white, the protein fraction of the egg:

"...one group of rats was injected with egg white, just to see how much stress this foreign protein would produce. Much to my surprise, egg white did not act merely as a stressor, but produced a very specific and strange syndrome. Immediately after the injection the rats seemed to be quite all right, but soon afterward they started to sneeze and sat up on their haunches, scratching their snouts with the forepaws. A few minutes later, their noses and lips became greatly swollen and red, giving the animals a very peculiar appearance."

Selye's description of the allergic effects of a foreign protein is a good introduction to food allergy. Human patients experience similar reactions to ingested protein as do the rats to injected protein. Selye compared the "stress response" to the "allergic response". If Selye had chosen to concentrate on the general theory of allergic response, rather than the whole body responses to non-specific physical stressors, our current vocabulary would probably use the word "allergy" instead of "stress". We are likely to discover in the next few decades that the many varieties of immune defenses (Allergy) operating within us are far more potent determinants of body-mind states than any number of non-specific experiential events (Stress).

A healthy child copes with a remarkable range of adversity and emerges intact, whereas a sick child cannot cope with the ordinary transactions of daily life. Allergy, as the adverse effects of immune defense, must be the most ubiquitous pattern of reactivity. We are reacting to specific physical agents in the molecular stream of food, water, and air. Even the symptoms of a cold or the flu are "allergic", since we mostly feel the adverse effects of the immune defense against the virus, and not just the action of the virus itself. All of the body responses that Selye investigated are implicated in allergic responses.

Biological stress (unpredictably changing body input) is reduced to a minimum by doing the same things every day. Food selection has the greatest impact on basic body states, and regularity in food consumption and correct food choices may be one the simplest methods of globally reducing biological stress. Nutritional programming strategies link body responses to cognitive-emotional events, to physical and molecular stressors entering body space from the environment.

1.0.6 The Core Diet Strategy

In my clinical and theoretical work, an entire system of techniques is considered to restore balance and order to the body of each patient. Diet revision therapy is an important subset of nutritional programming and shares the following therapeutic and preventive goals:

1. To recognize and eliminate adverse reactions to food, by any and all mechanisms.

2. To obtain optimal nutrient supply every day.

3. To balance energy needs dynamically so that mental status, body growth, and physical stamina are normal and stable.

4. To resolve compulsive, disordered, destructive eating.

5. To reduce chemical stressors - additives, toxins, contaminants, radioactivity.

6. To increase the protective effects of beneficial foods.

7. To resolve metabolic deficiencies or idiosyncrasies by compensatory nutrient programming.

8. To translate diet revision into food selections that are economical, practical, socially and esthetically acceptable.

Of the eight goals, the procedures for detecting and correcting adverse food reactions (especially food allergy) are the least understood and the most important to explore theoretically and practically. In other words, we seek and remove food problems before we do anything else.

Drs. Robert Good, Gabriel Fernandes, and Anne West, Medical Editor, Sloan-Kettering Cancer Centre, state in their review of Nutrition and Immunity[5]

> "We look forward to the time when the prophylactic and therapeutic potential of scientifically controlled diet, along with cellular, molecular, and hormonal engineering, may be realized and applied. Freedom of many disorders which have historically deprived us of our genetic legacy of a long and healthy life is certainly a worthwhile objective."

Ultimately, we may have the technology to monitor our body chemistry, in real-time process, and design specific, optimal nutrient intake for individual metabolisms. For now, lacking this technology, we can utilize our own self-monitoring and self-diagnostic abilities to better advantage. Better self-monitoring and adaptive self-directed changes in food and environment are the keys to successful diet revision and nutritional programming.

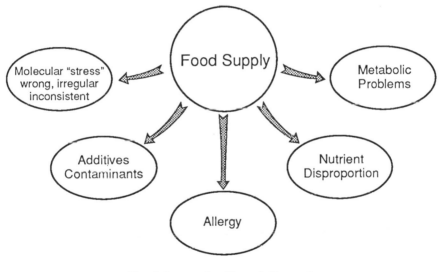

Problems in Food Supply

<u>Glossary Chapter 2</u>

AIDS	Acquired Immune Deficiency Syndrome
CD	Core Diet
CIC	Circulating Immune Complex
CURS	Chronic Upper Respiratory Syndrome
DH	Dermatitis Herpetiforms
DRT	Diet Revision Therapy
ENF	Elemental Nutrient Formula
FISR	Food Intake Symptom Record
IgE	Antibody: Produces immediate hypersensitivity
RAST	Radioabsorbent Test

Chapter 2

PATTERNS OF DYSFUNCTION

Human illness patterns evolve continuously as our environnment, food supply, and social patterns change. New foods, new eating patterns, increased food consumption, food additives, and environmental contaminants are the major forces of change in human disease patterns. Unrecognized food-related illnesses may have become the leading cause of human disease in affluent countries.

Children are especially vulnerable to problems in their food supply and suffer from wrong food choices, chemical additives, contaminants, nutrient deficiencies, and excesses. Newly emergent disease and dysfunction patterns in modern children, living in affluent societies, are poorly understood and may be denied by ill-informed professionals. It is a matter of urgent priority that food-related illness patterns be recognized, and investigated by well-funded international research.

Every human illness has at one time been misinterpreted and treated inappropriately. In this century, we have discovered and, for the most part, conquered infectious illnesses. Until AIDS emerged, modern medicine felt confident of its ability to conquer infectious disease. Non infectious disease is quite another matter - our success in understanding and treating all other endemic diseases does not compare to our ability to handle infection. Diseases that emerge slowly, with complex causation, are our biggest problems and do not obey the infection model - one cause, one disease, one treatment. Current problems have complex causation, with multiple variables not yet defined. A new level of sophisticated "systems thinking" and medical problem-solving is needed to deal effectively with modern problems.

I believe that food allergy is among the most important causes of modern disease. Food allergy is not a trivial, unusual problem. It is a common, profound set of body malfunctions that likely affects everyone to some degree or another. The manifestations of food allergy are prolific and cross the boundaries of many medical specialties. The versatility of food allergy and its ability to mimic many diseases challenges the basic assumptions of medical diagnosis and treatment which try to organize disease patterns into discrete, exclusive categories.

2.0.1 Medical Diagnosis: Categories vs Process

Many unpleasant experiences, in different patterns and sequences, tend to occur in every human being. From a physician's point of view, the dysfunctional experiences of the patient are interpreted as symptoms or indicators of disease. Physicians are taught to elicit patients' reports of specific symptoms in a certain order. This procedure is "diagnosis". The practice of diagnosis is deliberately designed to ignore a great deal of the information a patient provides. This diagnostic screening strategy serves us well in emergency situations, where triage is needed. We are used to dismissing certain patterns of dysfunction which we know from experience resolve spontaneously, or, at least, are not immediately life-threatening. The physician tries to organize a patient's symptom account into something like the following description:

> *...Crampy, periumbilical abdominal pain, associated with vomiting, but not diarrhea, which becomes steady and moves to the right lower quadrant in eight to twelve hours...*

This description is diagnostic of acute appendicitis. The medical diagnosis is completed by finding tenderness in the lower right abdomen over the appendix area, and finding an elevated temperature and an elevated white blood cell count in the laboratory.

Food allergy illness patterns, unfortunately, are not well-described in medical textbooks and are often not diagnosed nor treated properly. Many food allergy patterns are thought of as an ill-defined illness due to stress, flu, virus, colds, or are even dismissed as attention-getting or "psychosomatic" problems. I have been mapping patterns of illness in both children and adults with computer-assisted data bases. These symptom maps give us a clearer understanding of what is really going on in the community. Several food allergy patterns have become obvious in children, while others remain more obscure and need further research.

A child presenting with chronic nose congestion, cheek and ear flushing, a history of recurrent ear infections and tonsillitis, associated with infrequent attacks of abdominal pain and episodes of hyperactivity with temper tantrums is typical. Another child may present with recurrent "flu", fatigue, lymph node swelling and other vague symptoms - the doctors diagnosis may be "infectious mono" or "Epstein-Barr virus" or "candida infection". The proper diagnosis of these mysterious illnesses is "delayed pattern or Type III food allergy". If your doctor recognizes this pattern, (s)he should suggest diet revision - perhaps beginning with the exclusion of packaged and processed foods, milk, and dairy products from your child's diet. You would keep a daily food-intake-symptom journal with a return appointment in three weeks to review the results of your efforts. If the initial changes are not successful in resolving the problem, the Core Diet program would be the next logical step. With your physician's help, an ongoing healthy state should be achieved.

The diagnosis of delayed pattern food allergy is clinical - based on the history of illness and physical examination. Laboratory tests have not proved very helpful in making this diagnosis and skin tests, used to uncover the allergens in hay fever, also do not help in the diagnosis of delayed pattern food allergy. The case histories illustrated in this chapter should be helpful in identifying children with food allergy.

There are a set of typical physical signs which parents and teachers can easily spot and interpret. The allergic child has "shiners" - bluish-brownish discoloration around both eyes. The shiners may be accentuated by puffiness under the eyes, created by water retention (periorbital edema). The white of the eyes may appear pinkish or red from dilated blood vessels. Cheeks and ears may flush, appearing bright red to crimsom. Sometimes only one ear will flush, like a warning light. Nose congestion may present as mouth-breathing, sniffing, snuffling, snorting or snoring, or nose rubbing (sometimes known as the "allergic salute" - pushing the nose up with the palm of the hand until a crease develops across the skin of the nose). Nosebleeds are common in food allergy. The bleeding often originates from the front of the nose and is controlled by pinching both nostrils together for several minutes.

The lymphatic tissue of the nose and throat (lymph nodes, tonsils, adenoids) is the primary site of allergic response. It is not surprising then to find the tonsils and adenoids enlarged in an allergic child. Find and palpate the cervical lymph nodes ("glands") on either side of the neck. This lymphatic tissue is typically enlarged with food allergy and may swell dramatically to mark a food reaction. This swelling is often attributed (by mistake) to infection - either bacterial or viral. The allergic origin of the lymphatic enlargement is apparent after repeated or prolonged episodes. Antibiotics are often prescribed in vain and repeatedly without the physician realizing the diagnostic error (it is food allergy, not infection!).

2.1 Who to Treat with the Core Diet

The following summary of food allergy patterns and disease will help you identify problems in your children. All the following problems may respond well to Core Diet revision therapy.

2.1.1 Food Allergy Emergencies

Some food allergy is obvious. The so-called "immediate" reactions include mild swelling responses of lips and tongue and life-threatening anaphylaxis. Children who experience acute reactions repeatedly must follow a carefully chosen low-allergen diet and may not be safe eating out or eating packaged or processed foods. Generally the Core Diet approach is the safest and most convenient way to reconstruct a proper food supply.

The most obvious and dangerous pattern of food allergy is anaphylaxis, a life-threatening emergency. After eating seafood, nuts, or some other food a child may suddenly have trouble breathing, experience swelling of lips, tongue and throat, faint or collapse. Immediate treatment with injected adrenalin and life support systems will rescue the anaphylaxis victim. Acute severe asthma may also follow ingestion of an allergic food, and require emergency treatment. Vomiting and acute severe abdominal pain may also follow ingestion of an allergenic food within minutes. Itching, agitation, flushing, and hyperactivity also sometimes occurs within minutes of eating or may be delayed one to several hours.

2.1.2 Food Allergy as Chronic Illness

Food allergy is a whole-body disease and a lottery selection of disturbances may evolve over many years. In many older children, we can trace the illness pattern back to infancy with slow, intermittent emergence of symptoms over several years. In other children the illness begins abruptly and progresses rapidly without prior symptoms. A multisymptom and polysymptomatic pattern of illness means food allergy until proven otherwise.

The most common presentation of food allergy is that of a chronic, slowly progressive illness with many symptoms in many parts of the body. The illness may be mild and include nose congestion, headache, indigestion, flatulence, aching, stiffness and fatigue. The illness may be severe and present as intractable asthma, chronic diarrhea, failure to thrive, skin diseases, arthritis, urinary problems, hyperactivity, or learning disability.

A trial of the Core Diet will often produce dramatic remission of symptoms, even when parents and physicians doubt that food has anything to do with causing the illness.

2.1.3 Respiratory Disorders

The ear, nose, and throat are the most common target organs for food allergens. Congestion or inflammation of the nose (rhinitis), sinuses (sinusitis), and throat (pharyngitis) may be due to airborne irritants and allergens; however, food allergy may be the undiagnosed cause of these common problems. Food allergy is suggested by these respiratory symptoms: nasal stuffiness, snoring, increased mucus flow in nose and throat, ear-plugging with muffled hearing and ringing in the ears, recurrent middle ear "infection", recurrent sore throat, swelling of the neck lymph nodes (glands), chronic or recurrent cough, episodes of chest pain, "tightness", and/or wheezing with shortness of breath. Recurrent middle ear "infections" are very common in the first five years of life and may be eliminated by proper diet revision. Milk, wheat, and egg white allergy are the most common cause of respiratory symptoms, but any food allergy can do this. Ingested food additives - food dyes, sulphites, and salicylates - are also implicated.

Lung involvement, as a target organ for food allergens, tends to produce more serious and chronic breathing problems. Asthma, chronic bronchitis, and "pneumonia" are all possible consequences of food allergy. Often asthma is treated as an airborn allergy problem or as a problem unrelated to allergic processes and the possible role of food allergy is completely neglected! The mechanism of food allergic lung disease probably involves the wrong entry of food allergens through the digestive tract - food allergens interact with immune defenses in the blood stream and arrive in the lungs as immune complexes.

Chronic coughs may mean food allergic bronchitis with or without asthma. Food allergy patients are often given antibiotics repeatedly since allergic symptoms and infection symptoms are identical. Antibiotics may offer no benefits increase the risk of further allergic reactions. Many patients report long-term deterioration after repeated or prolonged antibiotic use. This apparent adverse effect of antibiotics has been blamed on yeast overgrowth, but the real reason is neglect to remove the real cause of the problem - wrong food!

Occasionally a child will react dangerously to allergenic food with an acute "pneumonia" (inflammatory swelling and edema of the lungs) and will require hospital treatment with adrenalin, nebulizers, oxygen, and steroids. Serious lung involvement will often clear if the child is maintained on an elemental nutrient formula.

2.1.4 Abdominal, Digestive Disorders

Food disappears into the food processor in the abdomen. Many symptoms appear as the immune sensing system in the gastrointestinal tract (GIT) reacts to the food passing through it. Children with abdominal pain, gas, bloating diarrhea, or constipation are suffering from food allergy until proven otherwise, and are prime candidates for the Core Diet. Milk and "high fiber" (whole wheat, bran) diets, recommended as staple food for children are often the cause of digestive problems.

Milk problems may be attributed to lactose intolerance and the milk-sugar enzyme, lactase, may be prescribed. *Milk allergy is a protein problem and is not improved by changing the milk sugar - often the diagnosis of "lactose intolerance" is incomplete or wrong and symptoms persist.*

Chronic diarrhea leads to malabsorption of nutrients, poor growth and development and increased risk of other forms of food allergic disease (eg. arthritis). Chronic diarrhea often will improve with the Core Diet program no matter what the underlying cause.

Another common symptom of gastrointestinal food allergy is rectal itching and/or burning, often with moderate to severe diaper rash in infants, and a perianal dermatitis in adults. Some girls experience chronic irritation around the anus and extending to the vulva and vagina. The irritation may also cause burning on urination. Yeast (candida) overgrowth occurs on the perianal skin, groin, vulva, and vagina. These common symptoms are related to the diet and fecal composition.

Candida growth is a consequence of food allergy, not a cause of it. Anti-fungal creams will clear the skin irritation, but lasting remission requires the removal of the original cause of allergic inflammation by proper diet revision.

Celiac disease (Gluten enteropathy) is the model of food-caused bowel disease. In this genetically-determined disorder, wheat proteins ("Gluten") are toxic to the bowel and produce inflammation with diarrhea and malabsorption of nutrients. The diagnosis is made clincially by typical history and confirmed by small intestine mucosal biopsy, which demonstrates atrophy of the absorptive surface of the small bowel. Far too many children have been denied proper diet revision therapy when a biopsy is reported as "normal". This diagnostic rigidity manifests the classic error of "treating the lab result" and not the child. All children with chronic diarrhea benefit from diet revision therapy, regardless of the biopsy result. Celiac children have increased bowel permeability and may demonstrate the whole-body effects of food allergy.

2.1.5 Skin Diseases

Children with food allergy often have skin disease. They may simply itch and squirm with little or no visible skin changes. The skin of the face, upper forearms, and front of the thighs may have a sand-paper surface with fine white to reddish bumps. Technically, these bumps can be called "perifollicular hyperkeratosis". I call them "milk bumps" since they are so common in cow's milk allergy, but they occur with other food allergens as well.

Eczema often appears on the face as patches of reddish, scaling skin. As eczema worsens, the skin becomes more itchy, red, thickened, and grooved, and may blister, weep, and crack. The typical distribution of eczema is on the face, behind the ears, on the fronts of the elbows, the backs of the knees, the hands, neck, and trunk. Hives are itchy, elevated, red blotches of varying size that appear suddenly and disappear mysteriously after hours to days. Other red rashes and skin bumps appear in various patterns during the course of food allergy - almost any skin eruption can be considered "allergic until proven otherwise". Eczema in infants and young children represents milk allergy until proven otherwise. Ezcema at any age should be considered a food allergy. Other skin manifestations of food allergy are itching, flushing, fine red rashes, hives, and acne-like eruptions. Psoriasis responds variably to diet revision therapy. Dermatitis Herpetiformis (DH), a less common skin disease, is another manifestation of wheat allergy and is a very slowly reacting process, often taking months to clear after diet revision, and days or weeks to recur after food challenge.

2.1.6 Migraine and Other Headaches

Children do suffer migraine headaches with severe pain, nausea, vomiting, visual disturbances, and light intolerance. Abominal migraine presents in a similar way, except the pain is in the abdomen rather than the head. The axiom that 80% of migraine comes through the mouth should apply. Most migraine suffers have true food allergy and are not just responding to biochemical triggers. Chocolate confections are a common cause of migraine, and normal food components - milk, wheat, barley, rye, oats, corn, eggs, peanuts, soya, almonds, cashews, oranges, and salmon - are all headache triggers. Migraine is a blood vessel disease, triggered by food allergens. In migraine's more serious forms, active constriction and, later, inflammation of the arteries supplying blood to the brain severely compromise brain blood flow and lead to symptoms suggestive of stroke. Major emotional, behavioral, and cognitive disturbances are common among migraine sufferers and inform us of the profound impact of this disease mechanism on brain function.

"Tension headaches" or generalized head-pain, associated with increased neck, scalp, and facial muscle tone and tenderness, and often associated with irritability and impairment of cognitive function, are also often caused by ingested substances and not "stress" or "tension". The muscle tension and soreness associated with these headaches is often an effect of the underlying biochemical cause of the pain and not a cause of it! Pop (especially colas), chocolate, eggs, cereal grains, milk, cheese, and ice creams are the more obvious foods strongly correlated with "tension" headaches in children.

2.1.7 Pain in Muscles, Joints, and Spine

Pain, aching, and stiffness are often produced by abnormal immune or biochemical responses to food components. Often children complain of leg and other pains, especially at night. Children's pain has often been called "growing pains" - utter nonsense! A trial of the Core Diet may be dramatically successful in alleviating these common symptoms. Children also develop inflammed tendon insertions - quadriceps (Osgoode-

Schlatter's disease) and achilles tendinitis are most common and may improve with the Core Diet and rest. Muscle aching and tenderness (myalgia) is also common in food allergy. There is growing evidence of allergy to food proteins, especially the glutens in cereal grains and the milk proteins. Increased intake of whole grains seems to be strongly correlated with increased incidence of chronic inflammatory connective tissue disease. The combination of abdominal bloating and/or pain with body aching and stiffness is diagnostic of milk and cereal-grain protein allergy.

2.1.8 Arthritis

Allergic arthritis is a definite entity which is often not diagnosed in children. Typically, an acute, painful swelling develops in one or more joints asymmetrically. Some children develop rheumatoid arthritis - usually with no apparent cause- and food allergy can be considered as a possible cause. Many foods and drugs can cause allergic arthritis - chocolate, potatoes, tomatoes, citrus fruits, almonds, wine, beef, pork, eggs, penicillin, and other drugs. Milk, eggs, and wheat remain the most constant chief sources of food allergens in arthritis. Arthritis is usually treated with salicylates or related anti-inflammatory drugs. All anti-arthritic medication can produce asthma or chronic rhinitis and a variety of allergic skin rashes. Gastrointestinal surface irritation, bleeding, and ulceration are routine problems of anti-arthritic medication. The avoidance of these complications makes diet revision a very attractive alternative to drugs.

2.1.9 Genito-Urinary Tract

Bed wetting is a common symptom of food allergy in younger children. Other more serious problems of the urinary tract may also accompany food allergy. Children with lower urinary tract symptoms, especially urgency and frequency of urination with or without burning on urination may be excreting irritative metabolites of food chemicals or mediator metabolites from systemic food allergic responses. Diet revision therapy should be considered when symptoms suggestive of cystitis or urethritis are recurrent and not explained by laboratory documented infections. In girls, recurrent vaginal irritation or burning on urination (vaginitis, urethritis) may have an allergic basis. The mucosal surfaces of the bladder and vagina should be thought of as similar to the nose, throat, and gastrointestinal mucosa, with similar allergic reactions to food allergens, circulating in the blood stream. If milk, wheat, and egg allergy can cause rhinitis, they can also result in vaginitis, urethritis, and cystitis.

The kidneys present a large filtering surface to blood contents and are vulnerable to damage by circulating immune complexes containing food allergens. The child's report of flank pain often imitates an attack of kidney infection or renal colic. Children with food allergy may have fever with flank pain and frequency of urination and are often invasively investigated and treated inappropriately, with no thought to a food antigen origin of their problem. Glomerulonephritis may sometimes be triggered by CIC's containing food protein antigens. The recurring triad of transient flank pain, blood or protein in the urine, and the presence of symptoms in other systems should suggest "food allergy". Treatment should begin with an elemental nutrient formula (Tolerex) under the supervision of a skilled physician before the Core Diet is attempted. Parents can use urine test sticks at home to monitor their child's urine everyday. With precise urine monitoring (blood, protein, ketones, pH), the effect of foods on kidney function can be accurately assessed.

2.1.10 Nervous System Disturbances

Children with food allergy present a bewildering variety of mental, emotional, and behavioral symptoms. They may present with symptoms as diverse as temper tantrums, nightmares, delayed speech, sleepiness, depression, dyslexia. The food-related disturbances of brain function may include any combination of disordered sensing, thinking, feeling, behaving, and remembering. Some children have such grossly disturbed brain function when they are fed the wrong foods that the diagnosis of many serious neuropsychiatric disorders may be considered (retardation, autism, depression, schizophrenia) before diet revision reveals the real cause. Epileptic seizures do occur as a consequence of food allergy. We are routinely and succesfully treating children with attention deficit disorder with or without hyperactivity on the Core Diet.

Eating disorders are an aspect of the food allergy complex. children with food allergy tend to be food specialists, eating a small selection of favorite foods and refusing other choices. They often prefer foods made with wheat and milk, and some refuse all vegetable foods. These children are also compulsive eaters, and crave sugar-containing foods. The Core Diet is an excellent program for children with cravings, compulsive eating, and associated emotional problems. Chapter 13 discusses addictive patterns and food. Chapter 14 further describes food-related mental, emotional, and behavioral problems.

2.2 Typical Case Histories

The following patient descriptions illustrate common patterns of food allergy in children. These problems will remain ill-defined-illness in most children, as long as physicians and patients alike are ignorant of the pathogenic process. Each child may have collection of symptoms in different body systems. The examples are chosen to illustrate the wide range of symptom patterns, the frequent association of physical and mental symptoms, and the association of learning disability with food allergy. Consult the end of the chapter for a summary of the diseases associated with food allergy.

The patient histories are diagnostic of the delayed patterns of food allergy, and all describe children who have improved with Core Diet revision therapy alone. All children who improve experience a return of their symptoms when they eat offending foods. We assume that a dysfunctional food matrix underlies the problem. The Core Diet, a rational problem-solving approach to diet revision therapy (DRT), tends to succeed when other interventions fail. No form of allergy testing determines their food allergy, but careful, insightful diet revision is effective.

Proper diet revision requires conscientious cooperation of the parents, children, and physician at a rational, responsible adult level. There are no tricks, gimmicks, drops, nor shots, and seldom are drugs involved in therapy. The path of diet revision therapy is not easy, however, since many lifestyle changes are involved. Proper nutrition is established as a safe-food list is developed by experience, and monitored by a Food-Intake-Symptom Record (FISR).

These case histories are adapted from my consultation notes and do not include a full description of the clinical course of each patient. There are many variations on the symptoms patterns described below. In general, we can say that patients with similar problem lists tend to do well on the Core Diet. The case histories present the initial problem description and all may conclude with the statement:

With appropriate diet revision therapy, using techniques to remove foods contributing to food allergy and to substitute less allergenic nourishing foods; and behavioral modification to ensure stability with new, more successful food selection and eating patterns; and nutritional methods to monitor nutrient intake to ensure adequate nutrition and techniques resolve metabolic problems; the behavior problems, learning difficulties, and illness patterns tend to resolve.

2.2.1 Vomiting and Failure to Thrive

A 12 month old infant presented with the problem of recurrent vomiting and failure to thrive. Mother was desperate, having tried many different formulas and feeding schedules with no lasting success. The doctors she consulted had started to blame her for the feeding failures. The infant started out on milk formula, which was associated with colic and vomiting. Several different brands were tried on doctors' advice. By 4 months, he had gained only 3 pounds and was switched to a soya formula which he tolerated for 4 weeks, but then all his disturbances recurred. Powdered infant feedings, fruit juices, and infant vegetable foods were tried, with little success. We switched him to Nutramigen, a hypoallergenic milk formula, based on hydrolysed milk protein, and he seemed to be accepting this well, with the addition of squash and sweet potato, 2 ounces/day. He has generalized food allergy pattern and will require a carefully supervised hypoallergenic diet for some time to come.

2.2.2 Infant Eczema

A 3 month old infant who was exclusively breast fed by a conscientious mother presented with severe eczema. His entire skin was red, blistering, and scaling. He was understandably irritable, often crying, and slept poorly through the night. Mother had been applying steroid creams to his skin and giving him oral antibiotics with little benefit. Her diet was unrestrained and she drank extra milk and ate generous amounts of yogurt and cheese on her physician's advice, to supply nutrients for lactation. In view of the infant's extreme distress, I advised the mother to go directly to a hypoallergenic diet, particularly with avoidance of all cow's milk protein. All medication was discontinued. Within two weeks of the mother's diet revision, the infant's skin was clearing dramatically, and he appeared to be much happier, sleeping through the night with only one brief wakening for feeding.

2.2.3 Temper Tantrums, Frequent Colds

A three year old boy presented with "continuous temper tantrums", sleep disturbances, and cold-like symptoms which had persisted since three months of age. He had received recurrent antibiotics for cold, cough, and ear "infections. His behavior grew progressively worse during his second year untll mother was desperate for help. In her words "nothing works - he cries, screams, protests, and fights all the time". Punishment was never effective in controlling his angry, aggressive outbursts. He was a fussy eater who would eat only bread, peanut butter, cookles, popsicles and he drank 3-4 glasses of milk and a similar amount of fruit juice, usually apple juice. He refused most vegetable foods. Physical signs of food allergy included allergic shiners, flushed cheeks and ears, nose swelling and enlarged lymph nodes in his neck. This child cleared promptly on the Core Diet, but required close supervision to prevent "cheating" on reactive foods (especially milk and apple juice) which produced prompt recurrence of hyperactive, angry behavior.

2.2.4 Screaming and Eczema

A two year old boy presented with excessive crying beginning at day 10 of his life, progressing to screaming fits in the second year. He was fed initially on a milk formula for 5 weeks - he cried incessantly, developed severe diaper rash with red, scaling skin on his cheeks and neck. A switch to soya formula was helpful, but symptoms returned after 5 months when mother began to introduce foods - wheat pablum, applesauce, apple juice, and yougurt. He began to have sceaming fits at the end of the first year with bursts of hyperactivity and sleep disturbances.

We encountered hypersensitivity at the beginning of the Core Diet revision and discontinued rice, peaches and pears - all triggered obvious flushing, followed by agitation and screaming fits. A portion of the ENF, tolerex, 200-300 Kcal/day was introduced to provide extra nutrients and food introduction was slowed to one new food every 10 days. He remained stable and well on a simple food list (carrots, peas, sweet potato, chicken, turkey) for several months before decreasing sensitivity permitted new food introductions.

Comment: Some children remain hypersensitive for several months and must remain on a simple food list to remain well. This child suffered extremely, and behaved like a terrorist when he was fed the wrong foods. On a limited safe food list he was happy, bright, and a pleasure to be with. Parents become anxious about limited food choices, but nutritional support with an ENF and/or vitamin-mineral supplements can ensure optimal nutrition with normal growth and development.

2.2.5 Migraine, Abdominal Pain, Sneezing

A nine year old boy presented the following problems:

1. Crampy abdominal pain of three months' duration.
2. Recurrent migraine headaches with vomiting.
3. Recurrent sneezing attacks.
4. Rectal itching, with burning discomfort.

He was breast fed for the first two years of his life, but had many infantile symptoms, including recurring colicky pain. He had intermittent symptoms since then, but appeared to have worsened in the past three months.

Mother described a 2 week trial elimination diet - milk and eggs were removed from his diet - which produced some benefit, but many symptoms did not clear. A food diary (on the milk-and-egg-free program) showed intake of grapefruit, orange, toast, honey, peanut butter, apple juice, lemonade, and cookies. He tended to be snacking on these trivial, and also allergenic, foods. His substantial meals were beef portions, potatoes, and a few vegetables. Mother had noted that on high fruit juice and citrus intake, he developed chankre sores in his mouth. He had continued to have headaches almost daily, with intermittent episodes of abdominal pain, which was most disturbing. Examination revealed: one ear was crimson red, allergic shiners (bluish circles under his eyes) were conspicous, the nasal mucosa (lining of the nose) was swollen, and the cervical lymph nodes were enlarged.

Comment: A "milk-and-egg-free" diet may remain a problem for a variety of reasons. This child's remaining foods were quite undesirable, and did not work out either in the short or long term. This example illustrates the fallacy of "elimination diets". The Core Diet is based on a different concept. The Core Diet assumes that complete diet revision is required to resolve illness. The problem with delayed patterns of food allergy is that increased permeability of the gastroinestinal tract admits "wrong stuff" into the circulation. Food and drink can be thought of as a body-input recipes which have to be matched to the gastrointestinal tract. If the input recipe fits, then food processing occurs normally without the problems of food allergy. Most children have problems with many foods and require fairly rigorous diet modification over a period of time to achieve good results.

2.2.6 Hyperactivity, Learning Disability, Rhinitis

An eight year old boy presented with:

1. Hyperactivity, and disruptive behavior at school.
2. Learning disability associated with attention deficit.
3. Chronic rhinitis with frequent "colds".
4. Moodiness, restless sleep, and nightmares.

This child had always been difficult and irritable. As an infant on a cow's milk formula, he suffered colic, sleeplessness, and screaming fits. He was troublesome as he became mobile; he was constantly in motion, destructive, accident-prone, and pugnacious. He often "attacked" his playmates with hurtful punching, kicking, and biting. Disciplinary measures seemed ineffectual. Poor adjustment to school was apparent immediately with apparent inattention, inability to sit, and loud, aggressive, destructive behavior. He spent two years in kindergarten, and then was moved into a special class where he remained a problem. Psychometric testing at the end of the third school year revealed above-average intelligence, superior spacial abilities, but poor language development.

Nose congestion and cough were common symptoms throughout his life and he had frequent "middle ear infections" treated with numerous courses of antibiotics and decongestants. Tubes had been inserted in his ears on three occasions with temporary benefit. He remained an idiosyncratic eater, specializing in milk, dairy products, bread, pasta, potatoes, meat, and apple juice. He refused all cooked vegetables, but would eat raw carrots. His favorite dinner was Kraft dinner with cheese, and Jello or ice cream. He had intense sugar cravings and defied his mother's sugar prohibitions. Mother would find cookies, candies, and chocolate bars stashed under his bed, and on one occasion he was caught stealing chocolate bars from a local store. He often complained of stomach aches and leg pains.

He did well on the Core Diet with remission of all his physical symptoms as long as he stayed with the Core Diet foods. His "addiction" to junk foods asserted itself from time to time with obvious return of symptoms.

2.2.7 Asthma, Diarrhea, Learning Difficulties

A 10 year boy presented with the following problems:

1. Asthma of four years duration, with episodes of coughing, wheezing, and associated emotional outbursts.

2. Diarrhea occurred intermittently, often with associated crampy abdominal pain. He had had several medical investigations for this, with no abnormalities detected. Medications had been prescribed to relieve pain.

3. Temper tantrums occurred several times a week. While this child was often pleasant and cooperative, he would have epsiodes of agitated, refractory behavior, often fighting aggressively with his sister and brother.

4. Learning difficulties at school were attributed to difficulties concentrating and to "attention-getting". He was often restless at school, talking inappropriately and acting "silly". His language skills were 1.5 years behind his grade level and he was receiving 5 hours of special help per week. Psychological evaluation had shown above-average intelligence, but low language performance scores and attention deficits.

The child's original diet featured 4-6 glasses of milk per day, Cheerios, grilled cheese sandwiches, Kraft dinner, apple juice, carrots (raw), beef, potatoes, hot dogs, whole-wheat crackers and cheese, ice cream, cookies, Coke, and the occasional cooked vegetable. He was described as a "picky eater" and refused to eat most foods not on his favorite list. He often ate compulsively (eg. several bowls of cereal at one sitting, or repeated servings of crackers and cheese).

He did well on the Core Diet (and has remained well for over 2 years). By Week 4, his parents stated there was "... a world of difference" and he was "...a joy to experience". The asthma, diarrhea, temper tantrums, and attention defict all improved together, showing that they are not separate problems, but simply different manifestations of the same all-powerful food allergy process.

2.2.8 Overweight and Tantrums

A 6 year old girl presented with weight control and emotional problems. Her mother stated that she was "bouncing off the walls at home...a whirlwind of activity...fighting, screaming, and explosive...". She was overweight at 80 lbs and looked conspicuously plump. Skin rashes with itching were common, and abdominal bloating was almost a daily occurrence. She was otherwise well, and was adapting to Grade 1 successfully.

This child responded promptly to the Core Diet and within the first week was asymptomatic with no further emotional storms. She lost 4 pounds in the first 4 weeks. She refused to eat rice, yams, or squash but accepted the other vegetables, fruit, poultry and fish. Initial weight loss on the Core Diet should be no more than 10% of body weight in an overweight child. We would rather wait for subsequent growth to normalize body weight. On the Core Diet, most children grow slender with excellent linear growth and reduced total body fat.

2.2.9 Belligerant Behavior

A seven year old boy presented with:

1. Recurrent abdominal bloating with pain.
2. Recurring facial dermatitis.
3. Episodic hyperactivity.
4. Extreme mood swings with aggressive, belligerent behavior.

His behavior disturbance was the most important concern of both his parents. He was frequently hyperactive, unmanageable, destructive, and extreme in terms of angry, aggressive, screaming behaviors. His parents apparently took him to Dr... who suggested he was allergic to milk and sugar. They eliminated dairy products, candy, pop and desserts, but otherwise continued feeding him as before. He improved somewhat with initial diet revision. That program apparently included expensive multi-supplements and his parents were not entirely satisfied with the results. They stated that he changed from a hyperactive boy to a moody child with more tantrums, crying, and moping. He had been a picky eater with strong sugar cravings and compulsive eating of sugar-containing foods. While he did not have dramatic manifestations of food allergy, his rashes and abdominal bloating suggested that possibility.

The behavior pattern described by his parents is one of the typical presentations of many of the children I see who respond to appropriate diet revision therapy. We, therefore, began a standard program following a hypoallergenic diet and introduced foods slowly to ascertain their effect. In short, he has done very well. His parents are both very positive about his improvement, but are now appreciating the difficulties of maintaining normal functioning. He has shown fairly marked hypersensitivity reactions to some foods, with conspicuous facial and ear flushing, nose congestion, and deepening of the allergic shiner effect (periorbital edema with blue discolouration from venous congestion). On a follow-up visit, his mother said that he was doing well, but occasionally he "cheats" and reacts, and his inappropriate behavior is usually noted by his school teacher who is alarmed by mild deviations from normal functioning.

2.2.10 Abdominal Pain, Learning Disability

This 6 year old boy presented with a chronic illness including several major problems:

1. Abdominal pain and diarrhea since early infancy. This child began life with colic, screaming fits, sleepless nights, and severe diaper rashes. He was fed a variety of milk-based infant formulas on the advice of at least three physicians for the first six months with continuing problems. Mother, on her own, switched to a soya formula at six months with improvement in digestive function. Currently he was having bouts of diarrhea with abdominal pain every 3-7 days, lasting 1-3 days. Otherwise, he was flatulent with smelly gas - his abdomen often appeared distended.

2. He had complained of headaches since age 4. He described pain in both sides of his forehead, and behind his eyes. Mother stated that she ignored the symptom on most days, but occasionally he got a very severe headache, with nausea and vomiting, and she kept him home from school.

3. Chronic nose congestion, cough, recurring middle-ear "infections", and repeated episodes of "bronchitis". The respiratory symptoms were apparent in the third week of life and had continued intermittently to the present. Some relief of nose congestion and cough was noted from 6-12 months after cow's milk was eliminated, but seemed to recur as he ate more solid foods. His adenoids were

removed at age 3. Tubes were inserted to drain his middle ears at age 3 and again at age 5. Currently he had a continuous stuffy nose, with snoring at night. He had had antibiotic treatment on 17 different occassions in the past 3 years (Mother kept the prescription receipts) for "middle-ear infections" and cold symptoms.

This child was often disturbed and difficult to manage. He had a high IQ, measured by a school pyschologist, and was considered a creative thinker, but had failed Grade 1 and was now in a special needs class. Attention deficit disorder with hyperactivity was diagnosed, and drug therapy with ritalin was recommended to his mother by a child psychiatrist. Mother was not keen on drug treatment, and after reading several books on dietary management of hyperactivity, started her own diet revision therapy with promising results. His diet had included large amounts of whole grain cereal, pasta, bread, 2 eggs/day, large amounts of peanut butter, jam, apple and orange juice, beef, potatoes, yogurt, cheese, and ice cream (mother had been avoiding milk itself, permitting about 1/2 cup per day in cereal). She had stopped all dairy products and high sugar foods, and had followed a "low amine" food list. The child had become calmer and slept better, with partial improvement in his respiratory symptoms; however, his digestive disturbances and headaches continued to occur, and he continued to have attention difficulties at school.

Comment. This child was quite ill and cleared completely on the Core Diet program. Selective food eliminations may reduce the problem list, but a definitive hypoallergenic diet, followed by careful diet redesign is required for complete long-term success. Many selective theories - the Feingold additive hypothesis, the sugar concerns, the amine or phenolic theory, the candida theory - have had popular moments, but all are inadequate to solve complex food problems. Diets based on the selective elimination of specific substances may be helpful since many foods, containing many ingredients, are eliminated. The Core Diet is the most comprehensive diet change ever used, and proves to be extraordinarily successful. We did encounter problems with some fruit introductions and soya products, and had compliance difficulties in the first three months. Follow-up in two years showed gratifying normality on the maintenance Core Diet, with rare symptoms occurrence, and normal school function.

2.2.11 Respiratory and Behavior Problems

A 4 year old brother and 6 year old sister presented with similar symptoms. The 6 year old girl presented with a history of chronic respiratory symptoms associated with fatigue, leg pains, loss of appetite with sugar cravings, and episodes of irritable depression associated with social withdrawal and low self-esteem.

Her brother presented with a similar respiratory syndrome; however, his behaviour problem was more severe. He began his life as an irritable crying infant with colic and has persisted in manifesting hyperactive often aggressive, belligerent behaviour. The chronic upper respiratory syndrome (CURS) is typical of the delayed pattern food allergy, and milk allergy in particular.

Both children did well with the Core Diet program. Mother's first follow-up report the statement " he is a happier, healthier child...it's like a dream come true...". Both children, however, have displayed sustained hypersensitivity and they are easily provoked by wrong food choices.

2.2.12 Pneumonia, Vomiting, Diarrhea, Learning Disabilty

This 11 year old girl was often quite ill. She presented with:

1. Recurrent episodes of "pneumonia" with 3 hospitalizations in 2 years, frequent antibiotic therapy, and chronic cough between episodes of acute illness.

2. Episodes of vomiting and diarrhea, often with crampy abdominal pain, at least 1-2 days/week. In the interim, she often complained of nausea, indigestion, and bloating.

3. Depression and fatigue plagued her. She had progressively withdrawn in the previous year, shunning friends and family, and had expressed low self-esteem, loss of pleasure and interest. Learning disability was a major problem and she had spent the last year in a "severely learning-disabled class". Attention deficit disorder and "dyslexia" had been diagnosed.

She was a picky, idosyncratic eater who seemed to cycle through specific food preferences - only pasta and cheese for several days, then scrambled eggs and toast for a few days and so on. She refused most vegetables. Her best average daily diet would consist of 2-3 bowls of wheat cereal, whole wheat toast, eggs 3-4 days per week, cheese or peanut butter and honey sandwiches, 2-6 cups of apple juice or fruit drinks, 1-2 cups of yogurt or ice cream, pasta with cheese, beef, potatoes, and a small portion of one vegetable (usually peas) per day. Mother avoided "junk foods" and provided one multi-vitamin-mineral tablet per day with at least 100 mg of additional vitamin C per day.

This child made a dramatic recovery on the Core Diet with remission of her major symptoms within 3 weeks of starting. Her parents and teachers reported her improvement with the following comments; "...overwhelmed by her improved state...", "...remarkable change...", "...consistently brighter, more cheerful, self-motivated...". Dramatic recoveries are the reward of the food allergist, and parents who persevere through the rigors of diet revision. Food allergies often present as serious, chronic illness, and often - tragically - are only treated symptomatically.

2.2.13 Cough, Headaches

This 9 year old girl suffered a great deal pain over a long period of time. She complained of headache and leg pains for several years, but, for at least 6 months, experienced generalized aching and stiffness with episodes of joint pain, especially her right knee. She stated: "My whole body hurts." Bouts of severe abdominal pain in the last three months had taken her to the hospital emergency on two occasions. Many tests had been done, but none were conclusive. Her physician was concerned that she was in the early stages of rheumatoid arthritis. Since she also had chronic nose congestion with red itchy eyes and bouts of coughing and sneezing, she was skin tested for inhalant allergies two years ago and was taking allergy shots once a week for house dust and grass pollens - no benefit was apparent from the shots, and Mother even thought they were making her worse. She regularly took antihistamine medication and Tylenol, as a pain reliever.

She had major learning problems, repeating Grade 2, and was now in a special education class. She missed a great deal deal of school because of illness, and also had difficulty concentrating. She tended to be passive and mild-mannered, and was well-liked. At home she was often tearful and expressed grave doubts about her self-worth. She was a picky eater with narrow food preferences. She mostly ate whole wheat bread as toast or sandwiches, drank 4-6 glasses of milk per day, ate cheese, macaroni, potatoes, beef, and prepacked soups (especially "Chicken-in-a-Mug").

Her improvement on the Core Diet was dramatic. Within 4 weeks, she was free of all symptoms and remained well as long as she stayed with the maintenance Core Diet. Her parents stated that her improvement was "...fantastic, she hasn't missed a day of school on the diet...she is a different child...". The last test from school that I saw was marked 62/70 - congratulations!

2.3 Summary of Problems Related to Food Allergy

The following list summarizes the great variety of disorders related to food allergy.

Haematology
Iron deficiency anemia
Low blood proteins
Thrombocytopenia
Eosinophilia
Thrombophlebitis

Gastrointestinal
Vomiting
Refusal of milk in infants
Abdominal pain
Sore mouth
Tongue burning
Aphthous ulcers
Sore throat,
Increased mucus
Gland swelling, neck
Swelling, lips, tongue,
Bloating, increased gas
Diarrhea
Malabsorption
Intestinal bleeding
Constipation
Rectal pain
Anal itching
Infantile colitis
Ulcerative colitis
Protein-losing enteropathy
Crohn's Disease

Respiratory
Nose congestion
Sinusitis
Chronic cough
Bronchitis
Asthma
Recurrent pneumonia
Frequent colds
Upper airway obstruction
Middle ear "infection"
Hearing loss
Ringing in the ear
Pneumonia
Heiner syndrome

Dermatology
Eczema
Hives
Rashes
Itching
Acne
Flushing
Butterfly rash, face
Contact rash
Diaper rash
Photosensitivity dermatitis
Angioedema (swelling)
Abnormal bruising
Dermatitis herpetiformis

Hair loss
Psoriasis

Neurologic and Behavioural
Chronic fatigue syndrome
Insomnia
Migraine headaches
Tension headaches
Pain - undiagnosed cause
Hyperactivity
Attention Deficit Disorder
Learning Disability
Memory loss
Epilepsy
Depression
Panic attacks

Musculoskeletal
Generalized aching, stiffness
Restless legs
Limb and Joint pain
Arthritis
Low back pain, chronic
Muscle cramps

Genitourinary
Bed wetting
Bladder inflammation
Frequency of urination
Protein in urine
Nephrotic syndrome
Vaginal irritation
Urethritis

Cardiovascular
Anaphylactic shock
Irregular heart rate and rhythm
Water retention - swelling

Miscellaneous
Weakness
Fatigue, lethargy
Ill-defined-illness
Recurrent infections
Failure to thrive
Sudden Infant Death Syndrome
Eye allergy, conjunctivitis
Uveitis

This diverse list of food allergy syndromes includes a description of food allergy developed by several leading authorities[6,7,8] Most food allergists would agree with the authors that the expressions of food allergic disease are diverse, profound, and not completely discovered. The best medical reference text is Brostroff and Challacombe's "Food Allergy and Intolerance".[9]

In these disorders, food is playing a causative or contributory role in a complex manner. Digestive, metabolic, immune, and biochemical properties of the food interact complexly. We do not have to specify exactly what the mechanism of adverse food reactions is to be successful therapists. I have successfully treated children with many of these disorders, primarily by diet revision therapy. Many of these allergic diseases cannot be diagnosed by easy tests and are not IgE-mediated. Allergy skin tests and IgE laboratory tests, RAST, FAST, MAST, or ELISA are often not helpful. Adequate diagnosis and treatment requires a trial of the Core Diet or similar hypoallergenic food program.

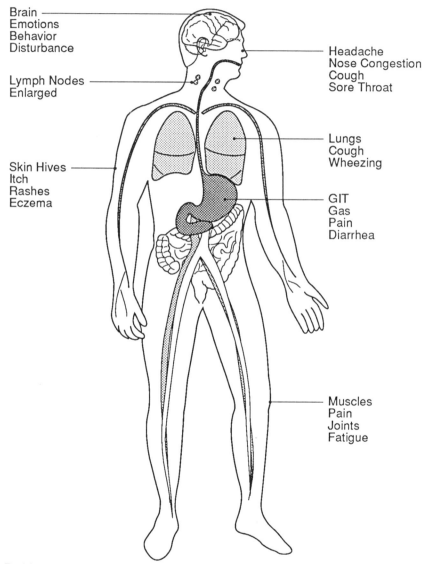

Brain
Emotions
Behavior
Disturbance

Headache
Nose Congestion
Cough
Sore Throat

Lymph Nodes
Enlarged

Lungs
Cough
Wheezing

Skin Hives
Itch
Rashes
Eczema

GIT
Gas
Pain
Diarrhea

Muscles
Pain
Joints
Fatigue

Problems Related to Food Allergy: Food allergens effect many parts of the body.

Glossary Chapter 3	
CSNA	Computer Scored Nutrient Analysis
DRT	Diet Revision Therapy
ENF	Elemental Nutrient Formula
ENFood	Brand of elemental nutrient formula
FISR	Food Intake Symptom Record
HYSENS	Hypersensitivity Phase

The Core Diet for Kids

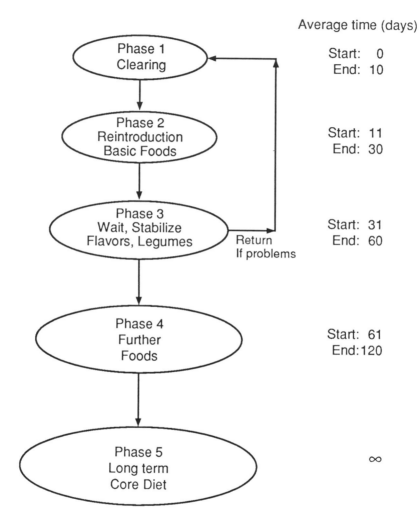

Average time (days)

Phase 1
Clearing

Start: 0
End: 10

Phase 2
Reintroduction
Basic Foods

Start: 11
End: 30

Phase 3
Wait, Stabilize
Flavors, Legumes

Return
If problems

Start: 31
End: 60

Phase 4
Further
Foods

Start: 61
End: 120

Phase 5
Long term
Core Diet

∞

Phases of Core Diet

Chapter 3

STAGES OF TRANSFORMATION

The best way to view your child's illnesses, emotional and behavioral disturbances is as a failure of adaptation - a mismatch between the biological properties of their body and the kind of food and environment we are offering them today.

Food-induced diseases are surprisingly diverse, and many different approaches to diet revision have been utilized in recent years. The Core Diet is a modern "state-of-the-art" procedure that have emerged from clinical experience and research in the past six years. The strategy of the Core Diet is similar to diet revision procedures used in clinical and research centres in many countries, and are well-supported by proper scientific research.

Food interacts with our bodies in a very complicated manner, and may produce dysfunction and illness in a variety of ways. Diet Revision Therapy is designed to solve several problems at once. You become the therapist and quickly learn to interpret your child's symptoms in a biological manner and make appropriate decisions about the right food supply.

Diet revision therapy has ancient roots. Medicine in different cultures over the past 2500 years has utilized diet revision as a basic healing strategy. We are invoking the principles of ancient Greek, Chinese, and Indian Medicine - treating illness by adjusting food choices to restore normal functioning.

The Core Diet includes primary foods, popular all over the world and, at the same time, excludes other foods that are staples in current North American diets. It may be that we are simply rediscovering a basic eating plan that better suits the ancient design of our digestive tract and metabolism. It may be that we are responding to modern problems of additives and contaminants in our food supply. It may be that we each too much of our

41

staple foods, especially meat, wheat, eggs, and milk. Whatever the underlying causes of food-related illness, the Core Diet program is based on successful outcomes in children and similar experiences in over 3000 adult patients. Core Diet food selection is success-oriented, and has no other basis in taste, preference, or ideology.

When you begin diet revision, you have only problems and doubt. Your task is to replace problems with solutions. As you begin, you really do not know what the solutions will be. You may compare the experience to traveling in a strange country - but you do have a map (the Core Diet instructions). Many other parents have successfully travelled down this path and we know the terrain quite well. The basic problem is that each child has individual needs. The task is to find the best fit of food choices with your child's special biological requirements. You observe your child's responses every day, and decide which foods cause trouble and which foods are okay.

3.0.1 Stop the Input of Molecular Nonsense

Our diets are complicated by many foods and beverages not essential to good nutrition. Therapeutic diets reduce or eliminate most of these complications. Candies, pop, gum, Jello, Kool-Aid, chocolate, cocoa, and all "junk foods" are rather obvious problems that we avoid.

Most bottled or packaged beverages, fast-foods and reward-foods present too many problems to remain in our diet program. Packaged and canned soups have not been well-tolerated. We are avoiding chemical additives in foods, and this means avoidance of most manufactured, packaged, processed food products on the supermarket shelves. Processed meats, ham, weiners, and sausages are avoided, for example, even when beef or pork are found to be acceptable foods.

Fruit juices and synthesized fruit beverages have proved to be a problem for too many children and we begin with complete exclusion of these drinks.

Salt is permitted in modest quantities. Sugar, by itself, is not responsible for symptom production; however, too much sugar triggers cravings, compulsive eating patterns, and disorders children's rather delicate metabolisms. Sugar, associated with an allergenic food, seems to increase the severity of adverse reactions. Exercise moderation in the use of all sugars.

The health-goal is to return to a diet of simple, carefully selected, natural foods. Fresh or frozen vegetables, fruit, poultry, and fish are the basic food choices. These are primary foods that allow us to reconstruct daily menus, with confidence of good nutrition, and stable life-long eating habits. For most children, a shift to meals featuring cooked vegetables is the most important change. The design of the Core Diet is based on experience solving the problem of food allergies. It begins with a basic low-allergenic food selection, and continues with slow sequential food introductions.

3.0.2 Food Allergy Considerations

Food allergy is a complicated series of body dysfunctions. Since there is no current testing method that reliably identifies the causes of food allergy, we cannot specify a short list of foods to avoid, and assume that everything else will function properly. We can assume that diets with low allergenic potential will be helpful in most children, and begin therapy with a "hypoallergenic diet".

Our first goal is to clear existing symptoms; therefore, hypoallergenic diets are designed to remove all of the common problem foods at the beginning of diet revision. This means the complete exclusion of dairy products, eggs, cereal grains, and other common foods, like peanut butter, citrus fruits, and bananas.

The first foods on the diet are chosen because of a low probability of adverse reactions. When symptoms are reduced, foods may be added back in an orderly manner to determine the limits of your child's tolerances. By monitoring your child's progress, you can identify recurring problems, and change the food selection to avoid them. If symptoms recur, you retreat to an early stage of the diet, even to the initial Phase 1 foods, for several days, to allow the disturbance to clear. The strategy is to custom-fit a diet plan to each child's needs.

3.0.3 Stages of Transformation

The Core Diet is a transformation technique. The potential for change in physical and mental state is great. There are typical experiences as children follow the Core Diet, with a range of individual variations and adjustments to the experiences. Most start the Core Diet in an adaptive, but symptomatic and dysfunctional state. Adaptation to the dysfunctional state involves many hidden adjustments and compensations. Each of us is influenced by a complex of lifestyle determinants, cognitive and emotional adjustments. In simple terms, we get used to feeling badly and adjust our habits and expectations to the state in which we find ourselves. Any worsening trend motivates us to change, but we may not be prepared for the the degree of change required to fully recover.

Therapeutic change disrupts the adaptations made thus far and is resisted at first by the adaptive mechanisms in our body. We should, therefore, expect some difficulties in changing our childrens' food choices, and prepare intelligently to cope with the problems encountered.

The stages of transformation can be summarized as follows:

1.   *Identification* of the need for diet revision therapy.

2.   *Preparation* for change including basic exclusion.

3.   *Phase 1: Clearing* program first induces withdrawal experiences - intensification of symptoms, cravings, fatigue, depression for 3-7 days, then clearing of symptoms begins with increased well-being in 3-10 days. 10 days or more.

4.   *Phase 2: Intitial Food Re-introduction* - slow, progressive addition of specified foods often with the occasional recurrence of symptoms, and decisions to delete specific foods from the Core Diet list. Patience, good self-monitoring, and decisions about the acceptability of each food are required. 4 weeks or more.

5.   *Phase 3: Stabilization* of a Core Diet with resolutions of emotional responses - self, family, and friends. A problem-solving approach to any symptom recurrence should result in a healthy asymptomatic state. This phase is complicated by increased sensitivity to foods, and "cheating" on the Core Diet may trigger major symptom recurrence. A recuperation strategy of retreating to Phase 1 foods for 1-3 days is implemented to clear new disturbances. A nutrient intake evaluation is desirable, with a long-term vitamin-mineral supplementation program implemented to assure optimal nutrient intake. New food additions are flavorings and legumes. 4-6 weeks.

6.   *Phase 4: Expansion of Core Diet.* If everything is going well further food introductions are appropriate to increase the variety of food choices and the palatability of meals. Often, new cooking methods and the use of substitutions (eg. baking with non-wheat flours) are important activities. 6-12 weeks.

6.   *Phase 5: Maintenance* of an individualized Core Diet as a successful strategy of self-maintainence over years to come.

3.0.4 Psychology of DRT

Approach diet change optimistically. We expect your child to be better. Often chronic symptoms disappear, and a happier, more productive child emerges. The improvement path is difficult and sometimes frustrating - our expectation of improvement supports the effort.

Family participation is important to children, who have great difficulty if their food is very different from everyone else's. With food allergy, several family members are often afflicted, but perhaps not to the same degree. If the whole family participates in Diet Revision, other family members will often benefit, even when no benefit is anticipated.

Diet Revision Therapy is kindly motivated, and intends no harm. We live in a pleasure-oriented culture, and often use food as a reward. Most of us grew up with a food reward and punishment system, and continue this tradition in the management of our own children. When we realize that a child's food selections may contribute to illness, behavioral problems, or learning dysfunction, we must adopt an entirely different approach to food selection.

Most children experience withdrawal of familiar foods as deprivation - a form of punishment. Our first task is to reassure your child that no punishment nor harm is intended when we restrict access to certain foods. We may say "no" to ice cream, for example, and explain that some foods may not work properly once inside their body.

Withholding some foods is a precaution, a protective decision, motivated by the best of parental instincts. It as is if nature has designed a cruel trick, with pleasure in the beginning of the eating experience and pain or dysfunction later. Your child may enjoy the taste and texture of chocolate ice cream - feeling loved by you for offering this reward - only to suffer abdominal pain, headache, or a burst of emotional disturbance minutes or hours later. Once we understand that the chocolate ice cream causes pain and other suffering, we no longer can offer that food as a pleasure. We are now obliged to protect the child as best we can from the chocolate-ice-cream illness.

Different food selection is a method of restoring and maintaining normal body function. Food is basic body fuel. I always explain to children that they are like expensive sports cars and that food is like "gas" and remind them that cars need exactly the right gas to function normally. A perfectly engineered car will be a terrible disappointment if you choose the wrong fuel at the gas pump. I tell them that our problem is that they were shipped without an operating manual and we have to start from scratch to figure out what the best fuel (food) is for them. The Core Diet is a fuel-design program that maximizes that chance of discovering right-fuel with a minimum of errors.

Our basic idea is that food must function according to the design specifications of the child's body - without biological problems! The no-problem criterion for food selection replaces all the other ideas of food selection - nutritional ideas, reward, pleasure, convenience, or tradition.

Each parent should review his or her own feelings towards food as entertainment, comfort, and reward. There are many emotional consequences of diet change. Often we have to re-think and change our discipline strategy. Food is no longer suitable as reward or punishment. Changes in food selection are naturally resisted, often with anger and tears. Children go through an emotional transition, comparable to grieving, as they recover from food-induced illness. Anger and denial are early stages of this transition and challenge every parent.

Understanding and compassion are the right responses to this natural resistance to change - never confrontation or punishment. Usually the major disturbance occurs in the first week of the Core Diet - the withdrawal period - and, with gentle, reassuring persistence, most parents can steer their children through the difficult period toward new foods and normal functioning.

Negotiation for the "best deal" follows anger and denial. Negotiation is a healthy adaptive reponse, and should be encouraged. Involve your child in meal planning, and inform your child clearly about the allowed foods at each stage of diet revision. Rewards can be offered for compliance to the rules of diet change. These are non-food rewards, especially your praise and pleasure at their accomplishment. A hug and verbal reassurance is always a good response to your child's distress. When praise and pleasure are not enough, try experience pleasures - family games, movies, sports, visits, more of your attention. Incentive rewards - allowance bonuses or presents - are desirable.

Your goal is to achieve a permanent, enduring solution to your child's problems. Today's difficulties are temporary, and will eventually seem insignificant when a new successful adaption is achieved in a few weeks.

3.1 The Food Allergy Complex

Common and serious diseases are caused by food allergy. These disease patterns are not well understood and often are not diagnosed or treated properly. One of the reasons for confusion is that there are *several different patterns* of food allergic disease. A simple, brief summary of two different patterns may help you understand the best approach to your child'problems. You should know, at least, that Immediate and Delayed Patterns of allergic disease are quite different:

Immediate allergic reactions are obvious, often dramatic, and are easier to diagnose and treat. The other patterns of allergic disease are not so simple and often elude detection. Delayed Pattern food allergic disease involves a bewildering array of symptoms; it underlies diseases as diverse as chronic rhinitis, middle-ear "infections", eczema, migraine and other headaches, asthma, inflammatory bowel diseases, and irritable bowel syndrome. Food allergy is also associated with mental-emotional disturbances. Disturbances of sleep, mood, memory, thinking, and feeling are common in the food allergy complex. Hyperactivity and attention deficit disorder often improve with the Core Diet program.

3.1.1 Type I Allergy Patterns

Immediate allergic reactions tend to be quick, obvious, and specific. Swelling reactions, itching, sneezing, coughing, wheezing, and hives are typical of Immediate-type reactions. Rarely, the reactions are severe or life-threatening. Hay fever, some cases of asthma, swelling reactions, and hives are all Type I allergy patterns. In the intestinal tract, Type I reactions include nausea, vomiting, abdominal pain, and diarrhea. This type of reaction is mostly produced by a specific antibody, IgE. The typical patient with has elevated blood levels of IgE and is said to be "hypersensitive."

Skin tests may be positive with this form of allergy and are sometimes helpful in diagnosis, although skin tests are never adequate to predict the complex response of the immune system to foods actually eaten. Negative skin tests for food allergy do not "rule out" food allergy. The elimination of specific foods or food groups are often used in the treatment of Type I allergy. The most common offenders are milk, eggs, wheat, corn, citrus fruits, peanuts, soya products, shellfish, crustaceans, some fruits, and nuts. Many foods can cause Type I reactions, but these are the main offenders. Most allergy diet books list menus and recipes for a single food group exclusion, like "milk-free" diets and so on. Advice to eliminate a list of foods identified by skin or other tests leaves most mothers in a state of confusion about what to feed their children. Unfortunately, selective elimination diets are of little use in most children with food allergy. The Core Diet is a better approach to diet revision in any type of food allergy pattern.

3.1.2 Delayed Food Allergy Patterns

Most food-allergic patterns are complex, internal problems that involve a whole body response to many different food allergens. The gastrointestinal tract may react adversely to the food passing through it. Often the entry of "wrong stuff" into the blood stream triggers symptoms within the first hour, and then a series of disturbances continues for many hours or days. You were probably not aware of the role of food in producing your child's symptoms because of the variable onset after eating, especially the long delays separating meals and symptoms.

The food allergic mechanisms triggered by the entry of "wrong stuff" create very complex patterns of disease or dysfunction. The Core Diet program is designed to reduce or eliminate many problems at the same time.

The most common expression of food allergy is *inflammation* in target tissues, which we feel as swelling, heat, pain, stiffness, and loss of function. Any disease described by the suffix "-itis" can be caused by food allergy. Delayed food allergic patterns tend to cause chronic disease.

Do *not* expect to be able to specify exactly what your child is allergic to, since the Delayed Food Allergy mechanisms are complex and variable, rather than simple and obvious. Unlike the immediate allergic responses, delayed food allergy is usually nonspecific with many different substances contributing to dysfunction and disease.

3.1.3 Tests for Allergic Disease

Medical diagnosis is based on the physician's knowledge of the patterns of illness. The diagnosis of food allergy is largely clincial (knowing the pattern of illness), and not the result of a battery of tests. Indeed, routine tests are often normal, even when food allergy is quite severe. Many of my patients have had numerous medical investigations without any progress in diagnosing their illness, nor any therapeutic benefit. Medical tests should be done to confirm clinical diagnoses, not to make them.

There is no valid laboratory testing technology available to define or specify food allergy patterns. Skin tests and RAST (blood) tests are *not* helpful in Delayed Patterns of food allergy, since these tests tend only to reveal Immediate hypersensitivity reactions, mediated by the antibody IgE.

There are promising laboratory tests, used in research studies, and eventually we may have more laboratory support in diagnosing and treating this disease. If you and your children have food allergy, you will often encounter ignorance about your disease and may not receive adequate medical support. Make your needs and views known to all suppliers of medical services in your area.

3.1.4 Invalid Tests

Unfortunately, there are invalid tests and treatments for "food and chemical sensitivity". There are several unproven "tests of food sensitivity" offered in various cities, usually at extra cost to you. Invalid procedures include cytotoxic tests, "muscle testing", "pendulum tests", "biokinesiology", "bio-electric field tests" (using Vega meters), and "electro-acupuncture" devices. These "tests" are not based on any known biology and are best described as "flaky" or "bizarre". Many blame the symptom complex of food allergy on "Candida" or "yeast" - this is not valid. Often, diet revision recommended by people using these tests will be helpful. This success does not validate the test, but does demonstrate the <u>success of diet revision as therapy</u> - ie. diet revision reduces or removes body input problems to your child's body, with subsequent improvement.

While the desire for specific tests and easy solutions is strong and understandable, avoid the casual advice of less discerning (more gullible) people you will meet. Your responsible, hard work in resolving your child's illness through careful diet revision is as necessary as it will be effective.

There are no tricks, short-cuts, nor get-rich-quick schemes that really work. Consult Chapter 12 for more information on invalid tests.

3.1.5 Post-Clearing High Sensitivity

The path of transformation, described by all my patients, is truly a journey of mythic proportions. The closer you get to your goal, the more difficult and demanding the journey becomes. The next phase after clearing is characterized by decreasing tolerance to food and chemicals in the environmental. The other way of describing decreasing tolerance is increasing sensitivity.

The term hypersensitivity phase (HYSENS) has been chosen to describe the phase of increasing allergic reactivity, appearing as foods are withdrawn, and often persisting for many weeks or months. During HYSENS, wrong food ingestion is more likely to produce an acute reaction: abdominal pain, headache, immediate sore throat, mucus flow or hoarseness, fever, temper tantrum are typical examples. It is as if low-grade chronic symptoms have been traded for acute dramatic symptoms of shorter duration. This newly emergent "reactivity" of a child in HYSENS is most convincing of the immunological mechanisms underlying the pre-existing disorder. It is likely that suppressed allergic mechanisms start operating again at higher gain - these mechanisms were probably suppressed by sustained doses of food antigens.

HYSENS is a useful phase, since reactive foods are now more readily identified when they are reintroduced. It is sometimes alarming to children who are beginning to feel well and indulge in a small treat, like a sandwich or chocolate bar, only to develop acute abdominal pain, headache or similar symptom. Heightened smell awareness appears with HYSENS and is associated with decreased tolerance for airborne chemical stressors - smoke, automotive exhaust, household chemicals and perfumes become more noxious. The decrease tolerance adds to the social burdens of the recovering child, since many environments are now unmistakeably obnoxious.

Abrupt changes in mood and behavior in the recovering child upsets parents, teachers and friends. Be prepared to explain the increased vulnerablitity of your child to physical factors to avoid another round of misunderstanding and resentment with people who fail to understand the major effect of food and environmental chemistry on the child's brain function.

HYSENS is a perfectly valid, fascinating biological phenomenon which needs detailed study. It is not "psychosomatic" or "neurotic". Your child is not "attention-seeking". An appropriate response to your child's increased allergic sensitivity is to offer more protection against food and environmental hazards. Be more selective about the school and social events they attend - you are protecting your children from unpleasant, undesirable, toxic, allergenic, and otherwise harmful people and environments. A newly emerging social awareness will support this appropriate, protective behavior. Schools, unfortunately, may be contributing to food allergy and environmental-illness with hot-dog days, vending machines, fast-food cafeterias and allergenic, toxic buildings. Discuss your efforts with your child's teacher(s) and ask for their understanding and cooperation. Adult tolerance for variations in the child's performance is essential to avoid inappropriate criticism and punishment.

HYSENS tends to stabilize after a few weeks and slowly increasing tolerance for more foods is experienced by many patients during the first year. A smaller number of children experience progressively decreasing tolerance in the first year. This is a difficult problem which requires expert management. There are many strategies to try to improve tolerance, but often a limited food list, supplemented by an Elemental Nutrient Formula (ENF or ENFood) and complete, calculated nutrient supplementation are the supports needed to stay well. The concurrent solution of environmental problems may also be required.

3.2 Clearing Methods

We begin the Core Diet with an attempt to "clear" major symptoms and restore well-being. Clearing involves a rest from problematic food ingestion, followed by careful refeeding. You have to begin from scratch and slowly build a safe diet by offering single foods in a slow, rational order of reintroduction.

Symptom and behavior monitoring remains the best available technology to evaluate the effects of different foods. No laboratory procedures, however expensive or elaborate, will give you accurate predictions of what foods will do after your child eats them. You have to try them out and pay attention to what happens over 24-48 hours. Your own food-testing, with careful record-keeping, remains the most important strategy in determining a safe, effective Core Diet.

There are three clearing options options:

Option 1: Clearing by Fasting.

Option 2: Clearing with an Elemental Nutrient Formula (ENF).

Option 3: Clearing on Phase 1 Core Diet.

3.2.1 Clearing by Fasting

Fasting is the most radical method of clearing and is not recommended for children. Some children inadvertently fast in the first week by adamantly refusing to eat rice and vegetables. If your child goes on a hunger strike, do not be overly concerned. Instead, await spontaneous clearing of their disturbance and offer foods patiently until they are ready to eat. The function of fasting is to *jump* out of the recursive looping of food reaction-intolerance-craving.

During a fast, or significant reduction in food intake, many metabolic adjustments occur and these may not smooth out right away. It is unfortunate that the first two to three days of a fast may be disturbed, but, by Day 4 or 5, most people experience significant clearing of their symptoms. Liberal water intake is desirable. The idea of an immunologically restful fast is to ingest as few troublesome or extraneous molecules as possible. The metabolic consequences of no sugar intake are also quite different. Once liver glycogen is used up, children convert to fatty acid metabolism. This is initially uncomfortable, as ketone bodies from fat oxidation accumulate and cause a metabolic acidosis.

3.2.2 Clearing with an ENF

There are many illnesses which require food abstinence without the difficulties or penalties of fasting. Nutrients may be supplied in a commercially-prepared formula which assures adequate nutrition, but avoids the allergens and other problems found in foods. An elemental nutrient formula (ENF) can be dramatically successful in resolving illness due to food allergy.[1,2,3] A variety of Elemental Nutrient Formulas have been designed by various research and commercial groups over the past 3 decades. A series of new ENF formulations developed by EnvironMed Research Inc. of Vancouver B.C.[4] are referred to as "ENFood" formulas. ENFood CF is the Children's Formula (CF), generally suited for clearing and nutrient supplementation purposes. Another product "Tolerex", usually marketed by the Norwich Eaton Co. as a product for medical use in hospitals, has been useful in treating children's illnesses.

If the beneficial effects of a properly formulated ENF were rediscovered as a drug-effect there would be front page headlines and universal rejoicing. An ENF does not cure all ills, but many people get dramatically better when they go off food and live on an ENF for 7-10 days. It is really not the ENF which "cures" the disease. The disease clears itself when the problematic body-input stops. The ENF simply supports nutrition in a reasonable manner while clearing takes place.

An ENF is a nutrient mixture with all essential nutrients in their pure form. ENF's are often prescribed by physicians to manage serious digestive diseases or to provide adequate nourishment when eating food is undesirable or impossible. If your child is ill enough from GIT dysfunction or other serious disease (eg. bad migraine, uncontrolled seizures, asthma, kidney disease, major behavioral problems) An ENF may promote rapid improvement and is usually prescribed for 7 to 10 days, sufficient time for major disturbances to remit. The elemental diet rest from food is followed by phase 1 of the Core Diet, supported by continuing use of an ENF.

ENFood is also useful as a nutrient supplement for children who refuse to eat adequately. Adding 500-800 Kcal per day of ENFood in fruit or soup bases will dramatically boost nutrient intake.

ENFood is a *hypoallergenic nutrient formula* that comes in a powder form to be mixed with water. It contains carbohydrate, amino acids, essential fats, and all the vitamins, and minerals needed to maintain your child's health. Because the diet is complete, there is no need to take any vitamin or mineral supplements. There are no common substitutes for ENF's. Diet powders, protein powders, soya protein or vegetable protein powders, and nutritional supplements (like instant breakfasts, Sustacal and Ensure) are, in fact, the opposite of an ENF, and cannot be used on a hypoallergenic program. Products containing herbs, "natural foods or plant materials" are similarly banned. All food preparations which contain large molecules, especially proteins (and hydrolysed proteins), are avoided on a hypoallergenic program.

7 Day Clearing Program: General Instructions The use of an ENF can be tricky. The following instructions are offered as a general idea of how you might proceed with an ENF. Detailed product instructions are required and professional supervision would be desirable.

ENFood can be used to "washout" problems before starting the Core Diet. Because ENFood is hypoallergenic and nutritionally complete, it will provide complete nutrition for the 7-10 days during which your child is not eating or drinking any other food, except for water. If symptoms are due to foods your child has been eating, the symptoms will be reduced or will disappear completely by the 7th to 10th day on ENFood.

Your child will miss eating solid foods while taking ENFood, but will not feel hungry after the initial food cravings subside. He/she may experience symptoms related to the withdrawal of foods eaten regularly. Withdrawal can produce headaches, fatigue, and other symptoms, lasting several days. The most intense withdrawal experiences come from high-sugar foods, fruit juices, and wheat- and milk-containing foods. Intense cravings are sometimes part of the withdrawal experience. Withdrawal symptoms usually subside in 3-5 days.

After your child clears on ENFood, start Phase 1 of the Core Diet. During food reintroduction, you can use ENFood as nutritional support, reducing the amount of ENFood he/she drinks as food intake increases. It is very important that you follow instructions exactly during the entire program.

Because ENFood will reduce or eliminate food allergy-related symptoms, any symptoms that appear while reintroducing foods will be due to the newly-introduced food.

If your child tolerates canned peaches and pears, these fruits will improve the palatability of ENFood. Some children prefer ENFood mixed with hot water, rather than chilled. If your child finds the slight odor (of amino acids) is objectionable, use a milk shake-type container with a lid so your child can drink the diet through a straw.

3.2.3 Food-Intake-Symptom Records

Keep a written food-intake-symptom record (FISR) as you proceed with the Core Diet plan. To be accurate, you should record all food and beverages in your notebook soon after your child eats, noting any symptoms or behavior problems as they emerge. The daily record should include a brief summary for the day which should be filled out every evening. A sample report appears at the end of the chapter. The daily report is written for your own information. If the cause of today's problem is not obvious, make notes to review for a later decision when you have more experience and more information. Symptom and behavior descriptions include:

1. The nature and pattern of any physical symptom or behavior disturbance you observe.

2. The degree or severity of disturbance, measured in your own terms (a O to 3 rating scale is helpful).

3. The time of onset and duration of symptoms

The daily journal will usually reward you with several benefits:

1. Your powers of self-observation will be sharpened.

2. Patterns of disturbance will become clear.

3. The correlation between food and beverages ingested and symptoms will be perceived and better understood.

4. You will develop a sense of control over the problems your child has. You will become more objective and feel less alarmed or threatened by symptom recurrences.

The Core Diet for Kids

As your child eats newly reintroduced foods, watch for disturbances during food introduction and following it (anytime during the 3 days). The interval between eating and symptoms may be minutes to hours. If symptoms occur overnight, for example, the foods eaten the previous evening, at dinner and for the evening snack, are all suspect. Once a food is suspected of causing a problem, it is temporarily dropped from the Core Diet food list, and added to a list of suspect foods which may be tried again later. The help of a physician skilled in food allergy management may be invaluable, since often proper symptom interpretation requires considerable medical experience and skill. (A manual to assist physicians in food allergy management is available in this series.)

You want to know if the trend is toward improvement or more problems. It helps to grade the severity of symptoms:

Level 1 - Mild: the symptoms are just present. You tend to ignore them if you are busy. Your child may complain once and then carry on or shown mild behavior changes - listless, tired or irritable, restless.

Level 2 - Moderate: the symptom bothers my child enough that you want to do something to relieve it. If the symptoms recur, you will take your child to the doctor. If behavior is disturbed, everyone around the child is uncomfortable, but it can be managed.

Level 3 - Major: your child cannot carry on with normal activities, and needs rest, medication, or another remedy. If behavior is disturbed, it is often unmanageable or outrageous, and all social activity is interrupted.

The weekly review of the food-intake-symptom record must answer the following questions:

1. Have your child's major symptoms diminished or disappeared?
2. What disturbances are left?
3. What apparent food reactions have occurred?
4. Have there been major exceptions to the food list?
5. What disturbances did the extra foods cause?
6. Are there other environmental problems?

Enter all foods suspected of causing reaction on a list marked Suspects...this becomes a list of foods to avoid for now; later, foods from this group may be eaten again and re-evaluated. You can use the food list in the back of the book to keep track.

No single bit evidence is enough to decide the final suitability of a given food. A score sheet approach makes sense and this is a technique we have used to evaluate food allergies. For example, we might look at a single patient's experience with one food, scoring its tolerance with different kinds of information:

		Score
Apples	History of eczema, itches; high intake of apple juice with cravings	3
	After five days on applesauce, and some apple juice, bed wetting recurred, with irritability and flushing, and an itchy rash appeared with skin bumps.	3
	Removed all apple products, rash cleared in 4 days, dry bed on second day, calmer with no flushing.	3

The maximum score of 3 is assigned when symptoms follow challenge with a food, even when the onset is delayed. A further 3 is assessed against the food if symptoms disappear when it is withdrawn. Safe foods have a 0 score; foods with 1-3 scores should be place on a "suspect list" and tried again in a few weeks. We often have mild reactions to foods in the first few weeks that subside after a few weeks have elapsed, making these previously "suspect" foods acceptable for occasional consumption (eaten once or twice a week).

Delayed patterns of food allergy are not obvious. We are dealing with a statistical analysis and not with one-to-one cause and effect relationships. You may not be sure about individual food reactions, but this uncertainty will not prevent you from making appropriate decisions. A similar degree of uncertainty confronts us with most other important life issues.

3.2.4 Symptoms

Immediate food reactions are easy to spot since the onset occurs minutes after eating and the symptoms are dramatic. Write down the specific food which caused it, where it came from, how you prepared it, and the details of the reaction. Consult Section 2 for more information on patterns of illness, and symptom production and interpretation.

We look for red flushing of cheeks and ears as one of the most obvious signs of a food reaction. You will notice this within minutes or a few hours at the most. Often an abrupt change in mood and/or activity level accompanies the flushing.

Often a child will become fidgety, silly, and inappropriate at the dinner table. This can be handled with a little insightful humor or the suggestion to leave the table and "burn off" the extra arousal with harmless activity. Any resistance to this "fun"-directed agitation may trigger an angry outburst. Do not be surprised if tears, temper-tantrums, or even outrageously inappropriate behavior follows the ingestion of certain foods. Our policy with abrupt behavior disturbances is to kindly, but firmly, take the child to their room or another quiet place for a cooling-off period. After, discuss the occurrence, its probable food cause, and preventive measures for the future.

Ask your child to report all symptoms - sore throats, headaches, indigestion, changes in bowel movements, and so on. Accept symptom reports objectively. Children do not usually invent symptoms. Show appropriate concern, but avoid over-reacting. Discuss the probable food causes of the symptoms and encourage your child to make appropriate decisions about their own food choices.

Do not punish children for their suffering! We avoid saying things like "...see what happens!...I told you not to eat it!... it's all your own fault...". It takes children and sensible mature adults a long time to learn how to self-manage. Be supportive. Be patient.

Other symptom responses to food are less obvious, more complex, and may not be apparent for several hours (even days) after eating. The delayed symptom responses are also variable.

It is unlikely that the same symptom patterns will occur exactly the same way twice in a row. Instead, we observe, over several weeks or months, a series of different, but related symptom complexes following food challenges. Occasionally, a severe response will follow several mild experiences; often no reaction occurs after a severe one. This variability reflects the complexity of food and its interaction with the body. If the cause of symptoms is not immediately apparent, we continue to assume that "food did it until proven otherwise". Review the food intake over the past 24-72 hours and select the *most probable cause*.

If we look at specific symptoms, like nose congestion, mucus production, pain, or itching, the underlying mechanism likely involves the chemical mediators used by the immune system. In general, we have noted that much of our suffering is the result of inflammation. The universal cause of pain is inflammatory events in various tissues. Inflammation means pain, redness, heat, and swelling. The lymph nodes on either side of the neck may swell and become tender. In the throat, expect soreness and increased mucus flow, while noting difficulty swallowing, speaking, and, sometimes, breathing.

Many discomforts arise from the digestive tract and are usually provoked by the food passing through it. Mouth sensations include tingling, swelling, numbness, burning, and, occasionally, little painful aphthous ulcers which develop on the gums or cheeks. Further down the esophagus, a deep burning sensation or aching pain may occur below the breast bone or upper abdomen. In the stomach and small intestine, a deep boring pain or crampy pains is most likely to inform us of difficulty. A sick feeling or nausea informs us of an adverse stomach environment and may precede vomiting, a defensive reflex which attempts to rid us of the noxious substances we have ingested. Food-irritants or mediated reactions in the bowel wall stimulate the muscular contractions of the bowel, rushing the contents through it. This defensive expulsion response is experienced as crampy abdominal pain and diarrhea. Inflammation of the intestine may impair peristalsis, and gas accumulates to produce uncomfortable bloating or distension.. As reactive food products pass through the colon, aching lower abdominal pain is experienced. As the problem exits, rectal-anal reactions are felt as itching, burning, and swelling of the surface veins. Some children have loose stools and/or excessive rectal mucus and leak feces into underpants and sheets.

Beyond the intestine, a variety of whole-body disturbances are possible. Detailed food-intake-symptom notes will assist in sorting out the relevant factors later. Review your FISR once a week with the intention of solving problems that were not so obvious. If your child had unexplained symptoms during the week, or felt less well, then decide what body input was most likely to be wrong and delete it, writing a new menu list for the next week.

3.2.5 Quantitative Nutritional Analysis

The search for food reaction patterns, and food allergens in particular, is distinct from a nutrient analysis. Often with restricted diets, it is difficult to get balanced nutritient intake. After a Core Diet is established, a computed nutrient inventory in done in my clinic to assess the children's nutritional status. An accurate computed nutrient analysis is better than guesswork or third-hand opinions, suggesting all manner of supplements, herbs, and potions. Nutrient analysis requires looking up each food in lengthy tables, calculating totals, averages, and proportions - a time-consuming and laborious task, seldom attempted by dieticians. This task suits computers well and can be accomplished by measuring your child's food intake for 4 days and submitting the food list to a computing centre for analysis. A Computer-Scored Nutrient Analysis (CSNA) resolves all the questions about nutrient adequacy and should be obtained once you have achieved a stable diet plan. Nutrient analysis forms that ask you to check off weekly or monthly quantities of foods eaten by recall are not acceptable - the data is too imprecise to be useful.

A professional CSNA may be obtained from Nutridata (see the diet record and mail-in submission form attached to this book). If you are submitting information on the Nutridata form, be sure that your food list is complete for at least four days, and that you report all supplements taken (along with their specific ingredient list). You should measure and record your child's food on representative days, so that the results tell us about your child's average level of nutrition.

Before the Diet

I'm almost always sick

ear aches

circles under the eyes

Wheeze my asthma is acting up

I'm sick

sore joints

always tired having to take medicine

After the Diet

I'm barely ever sick

no ear aches

no circles under the eyes

I feel great!

my asthma is getting better

no sore joints

no more medicine

almost never tired

by Angela O'Neill, age 10

THE CORE DIET FOR KIDS

Section 2

**Instruction Set For
The Core Diet Program**

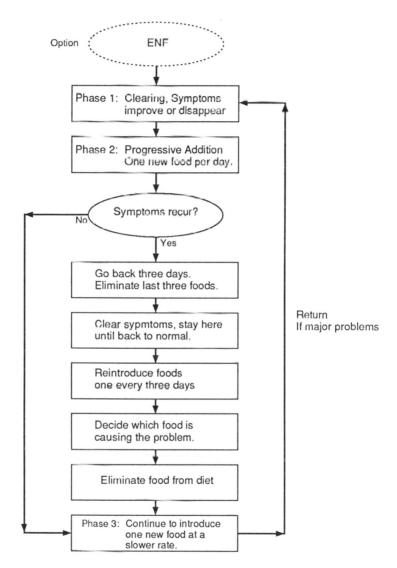

Core Diet Program

Glossary Chapter 4	
Clearing:	Disappearance of physical symptoms & emotional − behavioural disturbances
Withdrawl:	Period during which symptoms become worse, often emotional depression/distress occurs

Chapter 4

INSTRUCTIONS FOR CHILDREN'S CORE HYPOALLERGENIC DIET

This program is used for children ages 3 - 15. Older children may use the adult Core Diet method. Younger children may require modification of food choices, slower rate of food reintroduction and a different vitamin-mineral supplement list.

Diet Revision using the Core Diet is divided into several phases. The first two phases are the most important and most critical steps in diet revision therapy.

1. Phase 1: Clearing requires a minimum 10 days.

2. Phase 2: Progressive Food Reintroduction.

The outlines of Phases 1 and 2 are first described and then a detailed instruction set follows with food lists and cooking instruction.

Professional counselling and supervision are advisable whenever major diet revision is attempted.

4.0.1 Outline of Phase 1: Clearing Diet

Clearing refers to the disappearance of physical symptoms and emotional-behavioral disturbances.

The choice of foods and their order of introduction is determined by an analysis of the experiences of children who improved with diet revision. The best-tolerated, "safest" foods are eaten during the clearing week, establishing a basic "Core Diet" of staple foods around which you will build suitable menus for your child. Most of the foods on the Core Diet may be purchased at any regular food store

The Core Diet for Kids

Every child is different. Your goal is to custom-fit a safe, healthy diet plan to your child's unique needs. The beginning of this program is an approximation of a healthy, baseline food list. These foods offer a good start towards solving your child's health problems.

The amount of food you offer your child eat is determined by his or her appetite. Food refusal is common during the first week - do not worry, as most children show increased appetite in the second week and consume surprising amounts of vegetable foods.

4.0.2 Outline Phase 2: Food Re-introduction Plan

If your child is better at the end of the first week, we can assume that allergic activity has subsided and your child is tolerating Phase 1 foods. These foods are then kept as staple foods, and we begin to slowly reintroduce desirable foods. The slow progressive addition of single foods allows you to evaluate their effects and make decisions about their acceptability. The idea is to test individual foods or simple combinations, keeping track of symptoms or behavioral changes as you go along.

If your child is doing well, it is reasonable to add foods progressively, at the rate of one new food per day. If problems recur, we slow food introduction down to one new food every 3-7 days. Within 4 weeks, a reasonable "core diet" of basic safe foods may be established.

As you proceed, new foods are associated with slightly increased risks of symptom recurrence and you must watch your child carefully to notice return of symptoms or deterioration of behavior. If adverse reactions occur, decide what food is most likely responsible for the problem and drop it from the food list. Often you will not be certain, but our goal is to develop a perfectly safe therapeutic diet and, therefore, no doubtful foods are permitted at this time.

If major symptoms are encountered, progress is slowed until the symptoms go away; then, food introduction is resumed. It is important that you do not "skip ahead", trying foods before they are listed in the diet, nor should your child consume foods or beverages not listed. Also keep in mind that food mixtures act differently from food eaten in isolation.

While any food introduction and evaluation is underway, a diet record is kept. The record should show all the foods eaten and all the symptoms experienced (Food-Intake-Symptom Record or FISR).

INSTRUCTIONS FOR CHILDREN'S CORE HYPOALLERGENIC DIET

If you encounter a food on the introduction list to which you know your child is allergic, there is, of course, no need to test this food item; simply add it to your list of "unsafe" foods. If your child has had positive skin tests to specific foods on the list, but no previous experience of acute reactions, you may cautiously try offering the food. You would not do this, of course, if you already know that the food produces a major reaction, especially swelling, wheezing, hives, diarrhea, or abdominal pain. The occasional child has a life-threatening reaction to a food and must exercise extreme caution.

The more allergenic foods are not included in the food testing plan, nor in the Core Diet. The selection is empirically determined to achieve the best results for most people: for some, however, the choices will be less successful.

The meals you prepare will then be combinations of rice, cooked vegetables, simple salads with your own water-oil-herb dressing, poultry, fish, and some fruits. The principle beverage remains water, although now homemade vegetable juices and fruit juice can be tried. You reintroduce uncooked vegetables, adding salads and snack vegetables to your child's food choices. Unfortunately, there are more allergenic and digestive problems with uncooked vegetables.

Encourage your child to drink water - 4 to 6 glasses per day.

4.0.3 Cautions

While diet revision is probably the safest form of medical therapy, you should be aware of several important problems you may encounter with a major change in eating patterns. All of these problems can be resolved; knowing about the possible problems will help you to cope effectively with them.

1. *Withdrawal* from problematic foods often <u>increases</u> symptoms and distress for several days - current symptoms may increase in intensity or new symptoms may appear. Children often are quite distressed in the first 3 or 4 days, appearing tired, lethargic, or agitated. They commonly refuse vegetable foods and may be angry when you withhold the old favorites. Reassurance and patience is required initially. Tell your child that the "withdrawal" stage is often uncomfortable, but is short. It is sometimes necessary to keep children home for a few days to protect and comfort them as they go through the critical phase of withdrawal.

2. *Weight loss* may occur. Dramatic weight loss in the order of 2-3 pounds in the first week is mostly water - a positive sign that food allergic responses have stopped. Water excretion (diuresis) means increased urine flow, and may result in bed wetting for a few nights in younger children. Real weight loss, in the order of 1 pound per week, may occur in the next 2-3 weeks of diet revision. Weight stabilization occurs after several weeks on a hypoallergenic diet. Growth rates tend to increase once food problems are solved, so that initial short-term weight loss or food refusal should not concern us.

3. *Sensitivity to allergenic food substances* may increase in the first week on the Core Diet and continue for several weeks. The increased sensitivity seems to show that a previously suppressed immune "alarm system" is re-activated. As your child gets better, his/her body responds more quickly and dramatically to food allergens. Therefore, it is important that you are careful about making exceptions to the Core Diet food list, especially in the first four weeks.

4. *Nutrient deficiency* may occur with the unsupervised use of the Core Diet plan. Supplementation of both vitamins and minerals is required on long term hypoallergenic diets. A multi-vitamin-mineral supplement is taken initially.

   Symptoms during Phase 1 of diet revision may be due to:

   * withdrawal effects
   * metabolic disturbances
   * reduced caloric intake
   * cheating
   * allergy to Phase 1 foods
   * environmental problems

5. Symptoms during the first 4 days are usually due to withdrawal and reduced caloric intake. It is important to offer your child sufficient amounts of vegetable foods to avoid caloric deprivation.

6. With reduced carbohydrate intake, fat is used as a fuel with the production of acidic by-products; "acidosis" feels very uncomfortable for several days - nausea, weakness, fatigue, irritability, and headache are symptoms. Increased intake of

vegetable carbohydrate prevents acidosis. High caloric vegetables include rice, yams, sweet potato, winter squashes, carrots, turnip - these are highly recommended daily foods.

4.0.4 Vitamin-Mineral Supplements

A composite multiple vitamin-mineral supplement is desirable and convenient. Usually a multi-supplement and calcium are the two products you need to buy. The first approximation of amounts of supplemental vitamins and minerals for children ages 4-12 on a hypoallergenic diet is:

Calcium	250-500 mg	Potassium	200 mg
Magnesium	50-250 mg	Zinc	5 mg
Iodine	100 mcg*	Iron	20 mg
Fluoride	200 mcg*	Selenium	200 mcg*
Chromium	100 mcg*	Molybdenum	50 mcg*
Vitamin D	200 IU	Biotin	300 mcg*
Vitamin C	100-500 mg	Pyridoxine	50 mg
Folic acid	1.0 mg	Thiamine	5 mg
Niacin	5.0 mg	B-Carotene	2500 IU
Riboflavin	25.0 mg	Vit B12	50 mcg*
Vit E	100 IU	Panthothenate	250 mg

*mcg means Micro-gram or millionth of a gram; mg means milligram

An acceptable supplement must be "hypoallergenic" - without alfalfa, yeast, corn, wheat, soy, color, flavors, binders, preservatives, or animal glandular products.

*Avoid herbal mixtures:*It is usually *not* helpful to take acidophillus, digestive enzymes, bile salts, caprylic acid, garlic tablets, or other concoctions sold to improve digestion or immune function.

If you are concerned about weight loss, you may offer your child macronutrient supplementation with an elemental formula, *ENFood or Tolerex,* added to fruit or vegetable juice to provide a percentage of your child's daily nutrition. You should *not* use protein powders, milk-based formulas (Ensure, Sustacal), or formulas sold for weight loss purposes.

4.0.5 Laxatives

Constipation may be occur in the first weeks of the Core Diet plan, but is eventually corrected by increasing vegetable fiber intake. The best laxative to use temporarily is a bulk laxative - we prefer the plant fibre, Psyllium Mucilloid (Metamucil or Prodiem - choose unflavored varieties) at 1 teaspoon 2-3 times/day. This fiber is a natural gluten-free derivative of the husk of the grain Plantago ovata. The fiber absorbs water and increases the bulk of stools. The fiber probably also absorbs bowel irritants as it positively contributes to normalizing colonic action. Not only will it improve constipation, but it may also improve diarrhea. Occasionally psyllium mucilloid will cause abdominal bloating and must be discontinued. Do not expect a bulk laxative to produce the immediate action of irritant laxatives. Irritant laxatives, including cascara, senna, and castrol oil, are best avoided. Herbal laxatives of any description should be avoided. Herbal laxatives are mostly irritants; all plants contain potential allergens and toxins and may cause symptoms. I do not recommend enemas.

4.0.6 Monitoring and Records

It is a good idea to keep a daily food-intake-symptom record as you undertake the following diet revision plan. Describe each physical or behavioral disturbance. Note obvious signs of allergic reaction like cheek or ear flushing, itching, irritability, or sudden changes in behavior. Ask your child to report symptoms - headache, sore throat, abdominal pain, leg pain - and record these symptoms with the notations of time of onset, duration, and severity. Review the instructions for record keeping in the preceding chapter and read the problem-solving instructions following Phase 1 and 2 food instructions below.

The food choices for your first four weeks' menus are specified precisely in this hypoallergenic diet plan. *Any food or beverage not listed here should be avoided.*

4.1 Instructions for Phase 1: Clearing Diet

In older children (5-15) food introduction may follow the standard clearing diet plan outlined below with 12 foods offered during the first 10 days and one new food per day after 10 days. This is a rapid food reintroduction plan. Slower food introduction is necessary when children are ill, too young, very hypersensitive, or picky-fussy eaters who refuse to try new foods.

There are twelve common staple foods available during the clearing phase of the Core Diet which should last at least ten days. These foods are identified as "Phase 1 Foods" and are important for long-term eating success. A detailed profile of these basic foods is presented in "Core Diet Cooking".

The food list is limited in the first 10 days and no distinction is made between breakfast, lunch, and dinner. The food program resembles infant feeding. You provide your children the same healthy foods 3 or 4 times per day. The major change is to feed your child increased amounts of cooked vegetables - for breakfast, lunch and dinner!

4.1.1 Food List for Phase 1 Clearing Diet

Basic Foods	Zucchini	Thyme
Rice	Squash	Oregano
Rice cakes	Chicken	Basil
Rice cereal	Turkey	Parsley
Pears	Water	
Carrots		
Peas	**Condiments**	**Oils**
Peaches	Pepper	Safflower Oil
Yams	Salt	Sunflower Oil
Green beans	Rosemary	Olive oil
Broccoli		Linseed Oil

4.1.2 Standard Sequence: Clearing Diet - 10 Days

In older children, we often introduce foods in the following sequence:

Day 1 *rice, chicken, pears, carrots, peas, water*
Day 2 *rice, turkey, peaches, yams, green beans, water*
Day 3 *rice, chicken, peaches, carrots, broccoli, water*
Day 4 *rice, turkey, pears, yams, peas, water*
Day 5 *rice, chicken, pears, green beans, yams, water*
Day 6 *rice, turkey, peaches, carrots, green beans, water*
Day 7 *rice, chicken, pears, zucchini, peas, water*
Day 8 *rice, turkey, squash, peas, zucchini, peaches, water*
Day 9 *rice, chicken, green beans, yams, carrots, pears, water*
Day 10 *rice, turkey, squash, peas, broccoli, peaches, water*

You can alter the combination of Phase 1 foods if you like, but stick with these food choices. These foods are prepared simply with vegetable oils and basic condiments. Avoid any food that you know your child is allergic to. Stop any food that seems to trigger adverse reactions. At the same time encourage trying rice and vegetables, since most children do well on these foods.

4.1.3 Slow Phase 1

Younger children and children who are quite ill require a slower food introduction. We may have to introduce one food at a time and pace the rate of food introduction to the child's level of tolerance. We may, for example introduce one food at a time every 3 to 7 days to children between 1 and 3 years of age. The same food lists are used to direct food choices. Day 1 becomes week 1 and so on.

Occasionally a child is so hypersensitive that he (she) only tolerates a few foods from the Phase 1 list and a smaller number from the Phase 2 list for several months. If we encounter extreme HYSENS, we accept a small number of safe foods and add nutrients as an ENF and/or vitamin-mineral supplement. Often waiting at a modified phase 1 level for several weeks is the best strategy. Professional supervision and computed nutrient intakes assure adequate nutrition and optimal growth. Tolerance eventually increases, permitting further food introductions. There is no reason to hurry food introductions if basic foods + nutrient supplements are providing adequate nutrition.

Rice is the first food chosen, and may be presented as rice pablum, rice flakes (cooked cereal) or boiled rice pureed in the blender. Pureed carrots, squash, and yams are often the next foods offered to a young or sick child. The timing of food introduction is based on the child's status. Often we do better if we are patient and introduce foods slowly, being sure than no adverse reactions occur to one food before adding another. Often we organize Phase 1 foods into 4 groups, in order of priority of introduction. Establish Group A food first and then proceed through Group B and so on.

Phase 1 Group A: Rice, carrots, yams, peaches
Group B: Peas, chicken, squash, pears
Group C: Green beans, turkey, broccoli, zucchini
Group D: Salt, oil, flavoring herbs

4.1.4 Food Preparation - Phase 1

Vegetables: are the most important, most desirable foods. The vegetables must be well cooked during the first week of the diet. Steam-cook, bake, or microwave them. They may then be mashed or pureed (in a blender) to promote easy digestion. Soups made from pureed vegetables are also a good choice for easy digestibility.

Rice: This is the first desirable staple food tried. 1-2 cups of cooked rice per day will provide a caloric base - basic "fuel" for the day. Rice cakes and puffed rice cereal may be introduced in the first week. Rice cakes are substitutes for bread, crackers, and snack foods. Puffed rice, Rice Chex, or cooked rice cereal (rice flakes) are breakfast options.

Meat: Chicken and turkey, preferably breast meat is the first meat choice for. It is best to bake poach, or microwave poultry and fish - avoid frying. The poultry options can be dropped if you want to pursue a vegetarian menu.

Vegetarian Substitution: If you prefer to avoid poultry (and other meat) you can substitute another vegetable for the poultry option - combining rice with peas or green beans for each meal to improve the intake of essential amino acids; also add 1-2 teaspoons of vegetable oil. You may also add a small amount (1/2 to 1.0 ounce) of tofu to increase protein intake.

Fruit: Two fruits are selected during week 1: Canned peaches and pears. Cooked, home-canned, or commercially canned fruits (without sugar syrup) are acceptable. Choose a brand without preservative, sugar, or artificial coloring or flavoring. You may use peach or pear jam or jelly without food coloring or preservatives.

Vegetable Oils: Safflower, olive, linseed, or sunflower oil may be used in moderation (2-3 tspn/day).

Seasonings: Pepper, and light garden herbs - rosemary, thyme, oregano, basil, parsley - can be used for flavoring. Moderate <u>salt</u> intake is usually permissible.

Beverages: <u>Water</u> is the beverage of choice. Many children refuse water, craving the sugar of fruit juices. Be patient and encourage 3-6 glasses of water per day. Carbonated and soda water are allowed. Peaches and pears may be quickly converted to juice in a blender and added to carbonated water, if desired, to make a homemade soda. We avoid other packaged juices during the first 4 weeks of the Core Diet.

<u>Avoid</u> all other foods and beverages, especially hot spices, garlic, cinnamon, nutmeg, onions, tea (including herbal varieties) hot chocolate, chocolate, chewing gum, chips, pop, candies, all snack foods.

4.1.5 End of Phase 1

Your child's primary symptoms should diminish or disappear during the first 10 days unless you are unlucky enough to have problems with the initial foods (a 20% probablility).

Your child may complain about the lack of appealing breakfasts, and may experience hunger pangs with strong cravings, usually for a high sugar-foods. If your child has suffered from picky, fussy, or compulsive eating patterns, withdrawal tends to be difficult and the program may falter temporarily as you yield to demands, protests, or hunger-strikes due to withdrawal effects. Reassure your child that all will be well, be patient, and persevere. Small compromises usually get us through difficulties of the first week. Cravings fade away, hunger returns and a bowl of rice with carrots starts looking good!

4.1.6 Helpful Hints

You are undertaking a major change in you food selection and cooking habits. No one has found hypoallergenic diets easy to follow. Many families, however, cope well with the necessary changes and emerge with a healthier, happier child. The effort is obviously worthwhile. Resistance to diet change comes from all directions. Family cooperation is essential. Families who support an afflicted child by making whole-family core diet meals tend to succeed and often produce unexpected benefits for other family members.

Explain your child's problem to family and friends to avoid conflict, embarassment, and the inevitable "good advice", which is seldom helpful. Do not panic or despair when behavior problems recur - remember that "a food or drink did it until proven otherwise" and remove the culprit from your child's diet.

Use written instructions to family members, friends, and school. Be clear and specific about permitted foods - all foods not on the Core diet list are forbidden foods. Post a bold sign in the kitchen listing what foods are currently permitted and which foods are to be introduced during the next weeks. Children like certainty, and need reassurance that everything will be okay.

Try to be patient with food refusal and avoid confrontations or punishments regarding food. Do not force children to eat. Do not threaten.

Negotiate reasonably with your child - try to offer substitutes for missing foods, and alternative experiences to eating.

Offer rewards for trying new foods and finishing meals. Some parents offer a daily reward for diet completion - a star, token, or advance on a score board - with a cumulative prize at the end of the week. Treats, gifts, and rewards should not be foods - shift attention to activities and things. Reward your child with your enthusiasm and praise.

The real penalty for non-compliance is the illness and dysphoria suffered after eating wrong foods. Continue to explain the motive of diet revision - to reduce illness, and suffering -to help your child feel and function as well as (s)he can. Repeat the explanation often - 1000 repititions are better than 3. The choice of of which Phase 1 foods are included in a given meal is up to you. You may avoid a food you already known to be troublesome. Since rice is the staple, if your child seems to have symptoms from rice or refuses to eat it, try sweet potatoes, yams, squash, and carrots for vegetables with good caloric value. Millet or buckwheat may also be an acceptable substitute.

4.2 Monitoring and Problem-Solving

Take a problem-solving approach and monitor your child's progress on a daily basis. Symptom interpretation is an important aspect of problem-solving. Each child is a unique individual and many different problems may arise with diet revision. The following notes are offered as guidance. You may need professional help. Sustained cooperation of parents, children, physician, teachers, and other therapists may be required to solve problems as they emerge.

It takes a number of weeks to fully reconstruct your child's food intake with balanced, proper nutrition. It is important to be patient with children as they withdraw from old food habits, cravings, and compulsions. They often are genuinely distressed during the first week of the Core Diet, and you cannot assess their improvement until the second week. In the best case, improvement is obvious by Day 3 or 4 of the Core Diet, and food re-introductions cause little difficulty.

Approximately 60% of children clear uneventfully and experience an average of four obvious food reactions to the reintroduction of Core Diet foods during the first month. Unfortunately, they often have problems with the fruit options and are reluctant at first to eat vegetable foods. A subgroup of patients (about 20%) partially clear during week 1 of the Core Diet and require modification of the original food list before any new foods are added. Another subgroup of children (about 20%) do not clear at all during Week 1 of the Core Diet and reuqire careful re-evaluation - some of these children prove to be cheating and reveal strongly addictive behaviors that resist change (they cheat, lie, steal to get forbidden foods).

If symptoms are not improved by Day 11, the remaining problem should be solved before progressing to new food additions. Three options are available:

1. Review and revise Phase 1 food list. An astute parent will notice a food problem during the first week, but withdrawal symptoms and general confusion during such an abrupt change often obscures the origins of Week 1 symptoms. If you suspect any food, remove it from the list and continue with the remainder for 3-4 more days. If no further improvement occurs move top the second option.

2. If you cannot identify the offending food(s), remove rice, peaches, and chicken from the food list and continue eating the vegetables, turkey, and pears for 4 or more days. Try to boost vegetable intake to supply adequate daily calories. If this strategy seems to work, then start Phase 2 food introductions. Reintroduce rice and chicken after day 21-30 to re-assess their effect.

3. If all the above the food revisions are unsuccessful, a retreat to an elemental nutrient formula (ENFood) or even slow introduction of single foods may be required before you can produce remission of your child's symptoms. ENFood or Tolorox is a definitive clearing measure, but you should have professional guidance before pursuing this step.

You may encounter major symptoms beyond Day 10, but it is not necessary to abandon the Core Diet. Identify the probable cause and retreat to an earlier, more successful stage of the Core Diet. Some children have difficulty managing their food choices, and continue to fall victim to cravings, compulsions, and recursive-looping behaviors. These children will often resort to any lengths to obtain forbidden foods. Their "addictive" behavior does not promise a happy adulthood, and every effort should be made to help them out their addictive cycles at an early age.

Successful parents become good at monitoring their child and develop a flexible, adaptive approach. Often dietary advice implies that living is uneventful and easy, with few distractions from the business of looking after the needs of ourselves and our children. This illusion of an orderly, rational existence is misleading at best, and at worst, inspires real guilt and despair in those who believe others have an easier time of it. Since the Core Diet program is an exercise in scientific investigation, careful and systematic observation tends to reveal patterns of dysfunction and disease which otherwise remain mysteriously troublesome.

We all have preconceptions, prejudices, and blind-spots about ourselves and our children. We tend to resist change. We are tempted to rationalize our experience to avoid recognizing the need for major revision of our lifestyle, diet, and home environments. These blind-spots permit our problems to continue unchecked and obscure the origins of our disturbances.

4.3 Phase 2: Food Reintroduction Plan

The most important goal at this stage of diet revision is to develop safe, acceptable *vegetable* meals. <u>Try to combine 3 or more vegetables per meal.</u>

Continue to eat safe foods from the last week and add the new foods listed below. A suggested food introduction schedule follows the Phase 2 food list:

If a food reaction occurs after a meal with new food combinations, then the meal components need to be reviewed singly at another time. If your child feels unwell for any reason, postpone further food introductions until symptoms clear. Simply delay going on to the next day's food list until your child feels better.

Continue to keep a diet record to reveal any remaining problems and continue adjusting to the new food choices involved. Most mothers need to reorganize meal planning and food selection - ask for continued cooperation and help from other family members and friends.

Phase 2 Food List

<u>Vegetable Options</u>	Brown rice	Blueberries
Celery	Rice pancakes	Avocado
Cauliflower		
Lettuce	<u>Fruit Options</u>	<u>Fish Options</u>
Asparagus	Applesauce	Sole
Turnip	Watermelon	Halibut
Cucumber	Honeydew	Cod
Spinach	Cantaloupe	Tuna fish
Onions	Plums	
Brussels Sprouts	Apples	<u>Meat Options</u>
	Strawberries	Beef
<u>Rice Options</u>	Raspberries	Lamb
Rice bread		

Daily Meal Plans are based on selecting 3-4 cooked vegetables, rice, 1-3 raw vegetables as salad or finger food, selected fruits, and poultry or fish (see end of chapter for further suggestions). These foods are combined to make a variety of meals. Try to provide nourishing meals for breakfast and lunch by using dinner menus earlier in the day; vegetable soup, cooked rice cereals, or leftover dinner with chicken or fish, vegetables, and possibly some fruit are all good breakfast choices.

Consult the companion volume "Core Diet Cooking" for specific meal planning ideas and recipes. Continue the Daily Food-Intake-Symptom Record as an aid to monitoring and problem-solving.

4.3.1 Examples of Food Introductions Day 10-30

If we assume that the first 10 days of Phase 1 have gone smoothly, we continue to add one food per day to finish the second week. Our first choice is a white fish portion - a small amount first, perhaps 1 ounce. Next we are interested in more vegetable and fruit choices. We continue to serve foods from Phase 1, choosing rice (if tolerated) and 3-4 vegetables per meal.

Food Introductions, Completing Week 2:

Day 11	Sole
Day 12	Turnip
Day 13	Celery (cooked)
Day 14	Applesauce

Food Introductions Week 3:

Day 15	Honeydew melon
Day 16	Brussel Sprouts
Day 17	Cauliflower
Day 18	Rice bread
Day 19	Lettuce
Day 20	Asparagus
Day 21	Brown Rice

Food Introductions Week 4 +:

Day 22	Raspberries
Day 23	Cucumber
Day 24	Beef
Day 25	Plums
Day 26	Spinach
Day 27	Tuna fish
Day 28	Onions
Day 29	Avocado
Day 30	Cantelope

Several varieties of commercial *rice bread* are available. The ingredients vary widely and the recipes change often. Rice bread requires careful evaluation when it is consumed. In general, avoid those containing potato starch, as well as any other untested ingredients (yeast is a problem for some). Baking powder and baking soda are generally acceptable, although some children are sensitive to the trace amounts of wheat and/or corn found in commercial baking powder.

You now have enough food variety to cook meals with more attention to tasty mixtures and pleasing appearance. Vegetable mixtures can be colorfully arranged. The juices of vegetables cooked together with simple spices are delicious mixed with rice.

The style of Oriental cooking, blending small amounts of many different foods together into a complex and tasty mixture eaten with rice, is suitable at this stage.

If you have had no problems with cooked vegetables (eg. carrots, celery, zucchini, cabbage) you may try them, one at a time, as raw salad foods, if desirable. A homemade oil and vinegar or water dressing using safe herbs is alright for salads. Carrots and celery are good snacks if they are tolerated. Some mothers offer their children frozen vegetables as finger foods - frozen peas, carrots, or zucchini can be fun. Some vegetables are better cooked - especially broccoli, cauliflower, squash, sweet potatoes, and yams.

4.4 Further Problem-Solving

Problem-solving requires decisions to change the Core Diet program if symptoms persist. You make changes in your food lists and menus. Your goal is to be adaptable and flexible. *Retreat* to an earlier phase in the Core Diet menus if symptoms persist. If clearing was established during Phase 1, you can always re-establish clearing by going back to Phase 1 for 3-7 days. Avoid making "retreats" an emotional issue. Reassure your child again that the need to retreat is a normal requirement of food allergy management and does not mean that they have lost forever all their expanded food choices.

Remember that *no simple test can predict* complex responses to foods, since digestion, absorption, and metabolism are unpredictable, sequential phases of food processing that must evaluated by real-time, real-food, whole-system observation.

Remember also that *allergic effects are not consistent*. Do not expect to observe the same reaction each and every time the food is eaten. One convincing symptomatic response to a food is sufficient evidence in the early stages of the Core Diet to withhold the food for at least 3 weeks before re-evaluating. Our only goal in Phases 1 and 2 is to get your child better. We follow a cautious, conservative strategy, avoiding any food selection that suggests trouble.

4.4.1 Alter Timing, Portions, Frequency

Food allergic symptoms are related to the amount and frequency of food eaten, as well as the timing and circumstances of the meals. There are many variables to learn about. To solve recurring symptoms, we often have to alter food proportions, meal plans, or timing as much as food choices. Too much fruit, for example, often causes irritability, rashes, itches, intestinal gas or diarrhea, increased frequency of urination, or bed wetting. Reducing fruit intake to two portions per day and changing the fruit choice each day may resolve the problem. A child may refuse most vegetables as the fruit triggers cravings for more fruit or other sweet foods.

Solution: identify and withdraw offending fruit (eg. apples, apple juice); reduce the amount of fruit eaten - 2 portions/day is appropriate. Start a fruit rotation, assigning a different fruit to each day of the week:

	Mon	Tues	Wed	Thurs	Fri	Sat	Sun
Fruit	peach	pear	apple	melon	plum	pear	raspberry

4.4.2 Exceptions to the Diet Plan

If your child eats foods not on the list, simply record the experience in your daily record. Often unknown "cheating" will produce symptoms. It is important to understand the reasons for your child "cheating" on the Core Diet. Do not punish! Eating wrong food is inevitable. Everyone, young and old, makes exceptions, sometimes frequently.

As long as you can return to Core Diet foods, all deviations serve as random experiments and can teach you more about the way your child's body responds.

Sometimes the response is so severe, we vow never to allow it to happen again; at other times, there is little problem and we feel more confident about exceptions or treats. If a major slip from the Core Diet results in a burst of disturbance lasting several days, retreat to Phase 1 of the Core Diet and await symptom-clearing before you proceed to other food introductions. The *advance-retreat* pattern is the best way way to manage your child's food selection.

As we follow children over many years, we learn that every child changes a great deal, often gaining more tolerance for foods, but sometimes, inexplicably, losing tolerance. If you advance food options when things are going well and retreat, even to Phase 1 Core Diet foods, when you child is ill or disturbed, you will tend to get good results.

4.4.3 Important Management Principles

These are the most important behavioral management principles as you encounter compliance difficulties with your children:

1. Emphasize the positive. Reassure your child that diet revision will help them. You are trying to find "the right gas" for their body.

2. Accept early food refusals gracefully, but suggest over and over again that the Core Diet foods are **IN** and the other foods are **OUT** - simply as a matter of fact, and offer to try another method of food preparation and suggest "it tastes better".

3. Involve your child in meal planning and preparation. Have them prepare and taste food in the kitchen, and ask for their help in changing the food's flavor, taste, and consistency. The worst time to have a confrontation over food choices is at the dinner table.

4. Introduce your child to a vegetable garden - either real or through books with color photographs. Learn about and discuss natural foods. Encourage the whole family to participate in healthier eating.

5. If your child is strongly addictive, make every effort to remove not-allowed foods from the home.

6. Review compulsive-eating patterns in other family members, and hold a family conference, seeking the cooperation of everyone in reducing the opportunity and temptation of eating unwanted foods.

7. If the compulsive patterns are shared by other family members, then everyone should be following the Core Diet to achieve best results.

8. Remember that some foods are effective triggers of cravings and compulsive eating. Try to identify the "addictive triggers" that upset your child and arrange complete abstinence.

9. Be helpful and supportive. Avoid confrontation and punishment. Create a reward system for compliance with the Core Diet. Foods are never offered as rewards. Food withholding is never used as punishment!

10. Make sure your child is well-fed before going out into the tempting world. Instruct (with written food lists and explicit directions) relatives, friends' mothers, and neighbors to help you by not offering forbidden foods to your child.

4.5 Meal Planning

Plan your meals in advance. Vary your choice of "safe" foods so that your child is not eating the same foods every day. The variety and mix of the different foods assures your child will receive a spectrum of nutrients and also minimizes the negative effects of minor adverse reactions to single foods. Avoid serving the same fruit and meat choices every day. Continue to choose fresh or frozen foods. Continue to avoid packaged, bottled, canned, and processed foods.

4.5.1 Food Group Proportions

You should distribute the food groups in approximately the proportions listed below:

FOOD GROUPS	*PORTIONS*
Rice, Rice Products	*2-3/day*
Vegetables Cooked	*4-6/day*
Vegetables Uncooked	*3-4/day*
Fruit	*2/day*
Meat, Poultry, Fish, Tofu	*1-2/day*
Vegetable Oil	*1-3 tsp/day*
Water	*1 litre/day*

4.5.2 The 2/3 Rules

An adequate diet plan consists of 3 to 4 balanced meals per day. The actual amount of food eaten should be determined by your child's appetite, which, we hope, will work in a more balanced and physiological manner. It is important for your child to eat properly-prepared, well-balanced meals early in his/her activity day.

Three simple 2/3 rules help us select and distribute foods on the Core Diet:

1. Vegetable foods (including rice, rice products, or other grain alternatives) should account for two thirds (2/3) of your child's daily calories.

2. Cook approximately 2/3 of your vegetable foods and let your child eat the rest as fresh, raw salad or snack vegetables. If your child has persisting digestive difficulties, he/she may not tolerate raw vegetables.

3. About 2/3 of daily calories should be eaten by late afternoon (or within 8 hours of waking). Breakfast and lunch are important meals.

4.5.3 Breakfast

The best breakfast meals involve "real food" in the morning. The 2/3 rule suggests more of our principle cooked meals should be eaten earlier in the day. The best breakfast is a properly cooked meal. Think of poached rainbow trout, wild rice, carrots, and a sprig of parsley. A bowl of cooked rice with 2-3 vegetables (eg. carrots, peas, green beans) is a perfect breakfast. Rice can be fried (ie. warmed with vegetable oil, peas, cubed carrots, and perhaps fruit pieces in a frying pan to make a delicious breakast - a little salt and pepper may be the only flavor required.

Eating only fruit in the morning may work well for some people and not for others. Fruit is not nutritionally complete, and its high sugar content will often induce sugar cravings. Fruit juices are traditional breakfast foods, but are not always suitable for children with food allergies. The citrus juices and apple juice *have not been well-tolerated*, in our experience.

You can take any fruit that has proven to be "safe" and create homemade juices, using a blender or juicer. Homemade vegetable juices are highly desirable. Raw-food fans would suggest eating only fresh raw juiced vegetables; however, for many children this would produce digestive symptoms and increased allergenic effects. To avoid these effects, you can make juices from cooked vegetables. Cooked vegetables may be pureed in an ordinary blender; add water to achieve the right consistency.

Cereal breakfasts include puffed rice or millet, Rice Chexs, Rice Flakes, Rice Krispies, millet-rice flakes, or hot rice cereals, moistened with fruit and fruit juice or water instead of milk. Soy milk is introduced in Phase 3 and is often acceptable as a cow's milk substitute, if tolerated. Some mothers make rice pudding using, for example, rice, vanilla, soy milk, and raisins (leave the cinnamon and nutmeg out). Remember that 40% of children develop delayed symptoms from soy protein, especially if they consume large amounts every day. You may have to ration the amount of soy products in your child's diet to stay below a safe dose-frequency threshold.

Breakfast can be leftovers from the previous evening's dinner, perhaps mixed with fruit and warmed in the microwave. Why not have soup, salad, or stew in the morning? All over the world, for centuries, a single food pot would contain a soup-stew made of all available foods, simmering and available for every meal.

4.5.4 Lunch

Lunch should be based, if possible, on dinner menus - a full-course cooked meal is preferred. Often your child requires a lunch to take to school. A Core Diet soup, a salad, and rice cakes can easily prepared at home and taken in a warm food thermos. Lunch away from home may be cold chicken/turkey, salad (if you keep the dressing separate, the salad remains crisper), carrot sticks, rice cakes with a spread or jam, fruit, or any other relatively non-perishable food. Use a cooked-food thermos (food flask) and send rice and vegetables, hot soup, stew, or poultry or fish casserole.

4.5.5 Dinner

Dinner at home is generally the least difficult meal to create. A basic meal plan would begin with the choice of:

> *A rice portion.*
> *Cooked vegetables - choose a mixture of 3 or 4.*
> *Salad vegetables - choose a mixture of 2 or 3.*
> *A poultry, fish, or meat portion.*
> *Fruit.*

Vegetables can be chosen by their average nutritive properties. For example, choose four cooked vegetables using the following criteria:

1. One yellow-orange vegetable - tends to have a higher caloric value and is more filling - yams, sweet potatoes, winter squash, carrots, and turnips.

2. One legume - we begin with cooked peas and green beans, and later include dried beans, lentils, and split peas.

3. One brassica vegetable - broccoli, cauliflower, cabbage, and Brussels sprouts.

4. One (leafy) green vegetable - bok choy, spinach, and beet greens.

4.5.6 Weekly Menu Planning

Rotation diets have been advocated for many years as a solution to food allergy problems. Rotation plans can be complicated, difficult, and frustrating. Rotation plans do not work well enough to justify the major effort required to organize them. A regular change in food selection and meal plans is, however, a good idea.

The Core Diet replaces all other plans for food allergy management and tends to work best if you diversify your menus and alternate the safe foods on your child's list. The best way to alternate safe foods is to plan a week's menu in advance. List the safe foods you have established for your child and select the prerequisite number of foods from each food group. Assign these foods to the meals you are planning. The goal of your menu-planning is to balance food intake between stability of nutrient and energy supply, and taste diversity. Your child may eat staple foods every day if they are well-tolerated.

Your child will do best if you develop a standard menu plan for the week and follow the plan with few exceptions. Proceed now to Phase 3.

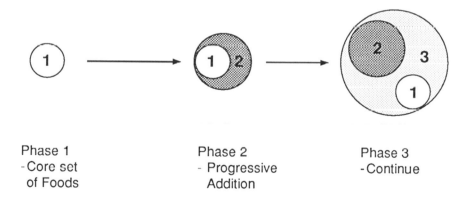

Phase 1
- Core set
of Foods

Phase 2
- Progressive
Addition

Phase 3
- Continue

Food Introduction Sequence:
- Within each phase you keep "safe" foods, thus tailoring your diet to your needs.
- You keep previous group of safe foods as you progress through the problem.

<u>Glossary Chapter 5</u>

Advance:	To progress forward in the Core Diet Program
Retreat:	To return to safer foods, recover and rest
RR&R	Retreat—Recover—Rest

Chapter 5

PHASES 3-5: FOUR WEEKS AND BEYOND

The Core Diet is a sequenced program of change, designed to reveal the origin of physical and mental problems. As you travel down the path, there are substantial rewards and some difficulties. Initial success with Core Diet revision is often dramatic; however symptoms do recur in each child with whom we have worked. Maintaining an asymptomatic healthy state requires a continuing effort to regulate your child's food supply.

The Core Diet program is designed to carry you through several problem-solving stages. After you complete Phase 1 - Initial Clearing and Phase 2 - Progressive Food Introductions, you are now ready to stabilize the improvements you have achieved, and solve any remaining problems.

The following instructions apply when your child emerges from Phase 2 quite well - major symptoms have abated and only recur when your child eats forbidden foods, not on the Core Diet list. The information provided in Section 3 of this book becomes more valuable as you experience the complex and fascinating details of diet revision therapy as a transformation path.

Phase 3 consists of securing the gains you have made thus far, problem-solving and then proceeding with further food introductions.

5.0.1 Stabilization

Following the successful reintroduction of basic Core Diet foods, we usually pause to practice eating from the new foods list. We also pause to solve any remaining problems that your child may experience. The idea is to stabilize a new healthier mode of functioning before making food selection more complex. Stability involves practicing and accepting Core Diet eating.

You may have problems making Core Diet meals interesting, and eating out is difficult. Your child may continue to have cravings for forbidden foods, and on some days may feel despondent with the thought that familiar eating "pleasures" may never be available again. We never say "never", so reassure your child that you are on his (her) side and just want them to feel as good as possible. We are trading some of the entertainment value of food for good biological functioning. You will try to find more replacements for old food pleasures in the next few weeks.

The goals for the next 4 weeks are:

1. To continue eating foods successfully introduced thus far, with the addition of a few more condiments as long as they are well tolerated.

2. To practice new cooking techniques - a more vegetarian-style cooking is often the most important new approach. This may involve wok-cooking, experimentation with soups, vegetable stews, rice dishes, salads and homemade salad dressings, rice-arrowroot flour baking, and so on. The companion volume "Core Diet Cooking" will be a valuable aid to meal planning and preparation.

3. To develop standard menus for each day of the week. Bigger, better breakfasts and lunches are usually required, using all food choices on the Core Diet. Lunch should become the big meal of the day, although a robust soup, salad, and rice cakes will do if you are rushed.

4. To continue careful self-monitoring of your child. Continue the daily food-intake-symptom journal. You will need to practice monitoring your child's progress every day, so that if symptoms recur you can try to identify the cause and correct the problem.

5. Often other recovery techniques, including remedial education, counselling for behavioral modification, and renewed involvement in play, sports, and other physical activities should be instituted at this time.

Our most important problem-solving rule is - food did it until proven otherwise.

You will likely discover that symptom responses are variable - some foods will prove perfectly safe and acceptable every day in any amount, and other foods will bother your child if eaten too much or too often or too fast or in combination with certain other foods. Your child's body works in a complex manner, and it is your task to tune-in to how your child feels so that your decisions about food will produce good results. Note-keeping is a very important part of this self-education process.

5.0.2 Behavioral Rules

Continue your policy of protecting your child from wrong foods and adverse environments. Remember that irritable, "hyper" or depressed behavior signals a food reaction until proven otherwise. Offer continuing encouragement and rewards for good compliance with the Core Diet rules. Maintain a regular meal schedule.

Mealtime may be the only occasion when the family is together, providing a good opportunity for friendly interaction. Be sure to set aside proper, formal mealtimes and allow sufficient time to enjoy meals. Make a rule that mealtimes are for eating only and avoid distractions (do not watch TV, for example). Avoid contentious conversation at the dinner table.

Food will feel much better to you and your child if you are both relaxed and enjoying the experience of eating together. Never force your child to eat. Avoid conversation about food choices at the dinner table. Keep your child well-informed about his or her food choices. Post written menus in advance of dinner.

Never use food withholding as punishment. Never offer food as rewards. Reward children for eating the proper food with praise and non-food prizes.

5.1 Phase 3 Food Additions

5.1.1 Flavoring Additions

We try more flavorings, baking, and cooking techniques to make Core Diet menus more interesting. Wait until your child feels quite well and stable before you introduce other flavoring choices. Add new flavors to meals that have worked well before, so that it is relatively easy to determine if the flavorings have any adverse effects. Add one at a time, alternating a flavoring addition with a new food introduction.

Flavorings	Celery seed	Seeds
Vanilla	Marjoram	Sesame seeds
Ketsup	Ginger	Tahini
Soy sauce	Mustard	Sunflower seeds
Dill	Carob	Pumpkin seeds
Bay leaves		

5.1.2 Soy Products and Other Legumes

We also try Soy products which have great appeal as substitutes for dairy products and meats in vegetarian, Chinese, and Japanese cooking.

Infant soy milk formulas (Soyalac, Isomil, Nursoy, ProSobee) are complete foods, useful in cooking and occasionally as a nutritional supplement for adults who need to gain weight. You can use the canned infant formulas as if they were condensed milk, on cereals and in baking. Regular soya milk is more difficult to digest and may be further complicated by additives. Soy protein, unfortunately, is allergenic and produces adverse reactions in about 40% of my patients. Tofu is refined soy protein - a good food to begin evaluating adverse responses to soy. Often only small amounts of soy protein are well-tolerated.

Peanuts are also favored by most children. Peanut butter is introduced as a spread on rice cake. Unfortunately peanuts and peanut butter are highly allergenic and we observe many problems after this food has been reintroduced. Compulsive eating of peanut butter is common and must be avoided. If peanut butter seems okay, limit the daily dose to one ounce at the most - dish out the daily amount into a serving dish or plastic container and keep the main supply out of reach. Buy plain peanut butter without added oils, sugar, or salt.

Other legumes are nutritionally desirable, especially lentils and beans, but also have some allergenic potential and contribute to gas and other digestive problems. Dried beans need careful cooking. Avoid eating several legumes at once (eg. peas, lentils, soy milk, tofu).

Soy Products	Legumes	White beans
Soy Milk	Peanuts	Split peas
Soy Infant formula	Yellow wax beans	Kidney beans
Tofu	Lentils	Chickpeas
Tofu products	Lima beans	
Tofu ice cream		

5.2 Phase 4: Further Food Additions

After the Phase 3 stabilization period of 4 weeks of symptom-free, normal functioning, most children are eager to try another round of new foods. If your child continues to have recurrent symptoms for any reason, postpone this phase of food reintroductions until symptoms clear - retreat to a safer eating position, rather than making things more complicated.

Remember that foods are added now with the same care and concern that we exercised when first introducing foods into the Core Diet. You must be convinced that the new food is well tolerated before you keep it in your child's diet.

Allow at least three days per new food to give you enough time to observe and correct delayed reactions. We often encounter symptom recurrence as more foods are added to the basic Core Diet. It is better to err on the conservative side, retreating to a simpler food list if any symptoms recur and waiting longer before attempting new food introductions. The following foods have been the best choices for developing the advanced Core Diet:

5.2.1 Vegetables

More vegetable and fruit choices are always desirable. The following vegetables may be eaten as optional choices, possibly once or twice per week. Introduce one food at a time - no more often that one new food every three days.

Bok Choy	Bean sprouts	Parsnip
Cabbage	Potatoes	Turnip
Beets	Tomatoes	Kale
Leeks	Pumpkin	Kohlrabi
Chard	Radish	Corn

5.2.2 Fruits

Fruit options are often appreciated by children. Introduce one new fruit per week during Phase 4; for more of a treat use jams, jellies, fruit salads or desserts. We continue to experience a variety of problems when children eat too much fruit. Continue to limit daily intake to about two portions. Be cautious about fruit juices as well. Take the attitude that you must be convinced that the fruit and/or juice is perfectly okay before you keep it in your child's regular safe food list. Avocado is included as a fruit, although its nutritive properties resemble a vegetable. Avocado make a good spread for rice cakes and it can, of course, be included in salads.

Avocado	Currants	Mango
Pineapple	Nectarines	Papaya
Apricots	Blackberries	Orange
Cranberries	Cherries	

5.2.3 Grain Alternates

For baking, cereal grain alternates and substitute flours may be tried. *The exclusion of wheat, rye, oats, and barley remains a firm policy of Phase 4 Core Diet.*

Buckwheat	Cornstarch
Millet	Arrowroot
Tapioca	Soy flour

5.3 Phase 5: Maintenance

The success of the Core Diet in resolving dysfunction and disease can be maintained for the rest of your child's life. The changes that you make by thoughtful, conscientious management are not temporary adjustments that you abandon once your child is well. The changes are enduring new habits of eating and self-regulation. Our basic maintenance strategy is to always follow the custom-fitted Core Diet that you create as closely as possible - allowing treats and exceptions of convenience or necessity, if adverse effects are not too serious.

There are so many variables which decide how your child reacts to food. All you can count on is change - children change continuously and the food selection youp present them will change if you are doing a good job of adjusting to their changing needs. We are aware of cyclic changes in food tolerance. Many patients find that they tolerate more foods in the summer, or when they are happy, relaxed, and well rested. Conversely, parents report that their child's food tolerance drops severely in the winter, or if they are tired, angry, or infected with a virus. Short daily rhythms also effect us - many patients report little food tolerance first thing in the morning, and more in the evening. Others report decreased symptoms if they exercise right after eating. Our food supply is constantly changing. Environmental variables throw many unknown complications in our direction. We seldom know from where the disturbances come.

Our method of dealing with variations in children's food tolerance and variations in the food supply is a common-sense problem-solving strategy; Advance and Retreat.

5.3.1 Advance and Retreat

Advance when everything is going well. You can expand your child's food choices, allowing more treats and exceptions to a strict Core Diet. We advance toward variety, pleasure, and convenience when the opportunity arises.

Retreat to a safer food list when symptoms return to recover and rest. Cravings and compulsive eating are often triggered by wrong foods, and may lead your child back to a prolonged session with recurrent illness. The most successful parent-managers learn to retreat to the Phase 1 Core Clearing Diet to allow their children to recover and rest when they get into trouble.

The most efficient technique of Retreat-Recover-Rest (RR&R) is return to a clearing program - either an ENFood or Phase 1 Core Diet, or a combination of both. We have found that minor symptom recurrences will clear by skipping a meal and having an ENFood instead. Major symptom recurrences require an ENFood or clearing diet for 3-4 days at least. Once your child is clear again, advance to the full 4 week Core Diet food list for the next few weeks until he/she is stable again.

5.3.2 Beyond Core Diet Foods

The most radical feature of Core Diet food selection is the exclusion of milk products, eggs, wheat, oats, rye, and barley. The less radical but equally important exclusion of popular drinks, packaged, canned, and bottled foods continues to be a problem to many families. There is always a strong pull back to old food habits and the more typical eating patterns of the community. Children continue to be bombarded by food advertising. Peer pressure draws them back to fast food outlets, snacks, treats, and junk food. On TV and on the streets, they are trained for the dysfunctional drug culture that pollutes and damages planet earth. You are battling this barrage of negative programming, encouraging them to pursue healthier, self-responsible eating habits. Do not give up!

The long-term Core Diet policy is based on the goals outlined in chapter one. These are sincere, serious goals that require our dedicated effort to permanently change our habits. Our experience to date suggests that children who stay on their own version of the Core Diet do best over the long term. They do best in all departments- general health, school performance, mental-health, growth, body-build, athletics, and self-esteem.

What if we reintroduce wheat products - some bread or pasta, for example? Some children, especially after 3-4 months tolerate small to moderate amounts of cereal-grain foods. Some children get recurrent symptoms, food cravings, and behavior changes and must withdraw to remain normal. Milk products are even more likely to trigger recurrent problems and we are even more reluctant to suggest reintroducing milk. *Once allergic to milk-always allergic to milk.* That is not to deny small amounts of dairy foods as treats - an ice cream cone on a hot Sunday afternoon, for example, may be pleasurable and well tolerated. If it is not well-tolerated then find substitutes - Rice Dream or tofu ice cream, possibly a sherbert or Dole Whip will be better tolerated treats.

Consider the following policy for further food re-introduction:

If your child is doing well after 3 months consider introducing one grain portion 3 days a week. You might choose oats or oatmeal first or a rye cracker. If after 3 weeks you are convinced that there are no recurrent symptoms, especially digestive symptoms, fatigue, irritability, or attention disorder, then introduce a wheat portion 3 days a week - a portion is 2 slices of bread or 1/2 cup of macaroni.

If the wheat protion is well tolerated 3 days a week after three weeks, introduce one portion per day. Continue to emphasize Core Diet foods with rice and rice products (if tolerated) still the staple foods. Increase wheat portions to two a day after 6 weeks if your child remain assymptomatic. Decrease or discontinue all cereal grains if symptoms recur or behavior deteriorates and wait another three months before repeating the experiment.

You can assume if symptoms recure with wheat challenge that your child will have a life-long limit on the amount of cereal grains tolerated in his or her diet.

If you are tempted by convenience foods - beware! There are a lot of unexpected problems even with porducts prepared from "safe foods". A child may be tolerating home made applesauce, for example, but reacts with flushing, hyperactivity, and bed wetting when mother introduces a new bottle apple juice. Packaged fruit juices have been a special source of disappointment. Dried fruits also may bring unpleasant suprises. Of course, we look for products that have no chemicals added, but this is no guarantee that all will be well. Keep the number of processed packaged foods to a minimum and introduce each new product as a separate new food. Be sure that your child is okay before you include any product in your safe food list. If symptoms recur, automatically exclude all manufactured food products as part of RR&R.

5.3.3 Protecting Your Child

Children are often given food as treats or rewards without any thought to their biological needs. Too many people have frivolous and irresponsible attitudes toward feeding children. Many are ignorant of the serious effects of food allergy. Many deny the profound effect of adverse food reactions on behavior, emotions, and learning ability. Unfortunately we have encountered examples of this ignorance among professionals, who should know better.

You must be firm in your resolve to protect your child. Your task is to discourage careless feeding of your children, and to encourage proper food selection. We make a careful distinction between the immediate, but brief pleasure of a food in the mouth, and the hours of suffering that may follow the ingestion of an allergenic food.

Some children are good at saying "no". Others court temptation and need constant supervision, at least in the first few months of diet control. Some mothers have made special hats, T-shirts, or signs to discourage careless feeding after many polite requests of relatives and neighbors have failed.

Make an attempt to send alternative treats with your children when they go to a party. In planning your own parties, emphasize fun and games more than food, and offer non-food prizes. Some artistic mothers are good at making fun objects with cut vegetables, fruit, and toothpicks - a carrot/cucumber car is not difficult to make. There are many treats that fit the Core Diet specifications, although an extra effort is required to replace the readily available candies, cookies, cakes and ice cream (see "Core Diet Cooking").

If your child is visiting someone, send a written menu. Be explicit. Mistakes and embarassment arise from too little information. Prepare a short safe food list and have several copies made so that it it is easy to distribute your instructions to neighbors, family, friends, and school.

Traveling and eating out are the most hazardous activities for Core Dieters. When you travel, take your own food whenever possible. Carrots, celery, rice cakes, and fruit are portable foods. An ENFood is a safe, convenient travel food - blend it with fruit to make a quick, complete meal anywhere in the world. Be selective when you eat out. The cheaper, fast-food restaurants have rigid, mass-produced food choices with many chemical additives and synthetic materials. Avoid these food outlets. Choose restaurants which allow you to select individual food items. Often it is helpful to have simple written directions to give to the waiter or waitress. The following example is a restaurant note used by a parent; it was simply typewritten and photocopied on pocket-sized cards to hand out. Cooperation with this written request was generally excellent.

"My child is on a hypoallergenic diet. He (She) is unable
to eat milk, dairy products, eggs, and wheat (flour).

Please prepare vegetables steam-cooked without sauces.
Also please bake or microwave meat, fish and poultry
without breading or sauces.

Please avoid using sulphates on fresh vegetables and MSG
or tenderizers in soups or on food.

Thank you for your consideration."

If we become more specific and discriminating in choosing restaurant
foods, it will eventually influence restaurant practices and make it easier for
everyone with food intolerances to receive the appropriate consideration.
Good luck!

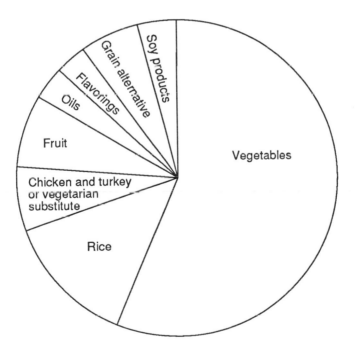

Example Proportions of Foods in Core Diet

Sample Food-Intake-Symptom-Record

Date: _____

Food	Morning	Afternoon	Evening
Symptoms	**Morning**	**Afternoon**	**Evening**

Comments:

1. List foods to be tested today. Mark a check in the appropriate box for time of day each time that food is eaten.
2. List symptoms as they occur, scoring them on a 0-3 scale (where 0 is no problem, 1 is mild, 2 is moderate, and 3 is severe.
3. Review today's FISR tomorrow and corelate symptoms with foods eaten, using the comment area.

THE CORE DIET FOR KIDS

Section 3

Concepts Supporting the Core Diet

**Advanced Lessons for Parents
and Professionals**

Glossary Chapter 6

AB	Alcoholic Beverage
DNA	Deoxyribonucleic Acid
ENF	Elemental Nutrient Formula
IgA	Immunoglobulin A(antibody)
IgE	Immunoglobulin E
IMD.E1	Immune Mediated Disease, Type I:GIT
GIT	Gastro—intestinal tract
NP	Nutritional Programming

Chapter 6

FEEDING POLICY: INFANTS AND CHILDREN

The biological fate of an individual is cast in the combination of mother and father's genetic codes. DNA encodes a developmental sequence which determines both the timing and pattern of growth.

Our first environment is the maternal womb. The growing fetus is fed through the maternal placenta, via the umbilical cord. The placenta is a selective boundary that separates the fetus from the mother, and she, in turn, separates the fetus from the dangers of the world at large with her own filters and buffers. The growing fetus should be isolated from the mother's environment by the placenta, but is not completely. We know that large molecules and even cells are exchanged through the placenta. From an immunological point of view, the fetus is sensitized through the mother to food and environmental antigens, and is born with some readiness to react defensively to the environment. The immunological response of the newborn may be appropriately defensive or may be allergic.

6.0.1 Breast-Feeding is Best

There is little doubt that mother's milk is the best food for infants. Human milk offers an ideal balance of nutrients and also contains a rich supply of protective factors which the human infant requires. Cow's milk is dissimilar to human milk in all respects. Although commercially prepared formulas, made from cow's milk or soya beans, have progressed over the years toward a more "human" composition by significant processing of the milk and addition of nutrients, these formulas remain inferior to human milk.[15]

Among the benefits of mother's milk is a generous supply of IgA, the protective antibody which the infant bowel lacks. This antibody helps to protect the infant from bacterial infection and probably reduces the entry of antigenic food protein fragments, reducing the incidence of allergy. Breast feeding an infant for six months or longer appears to significantly reduce the indidence of infection and food allergy.

6.0.2 Infant Nutritional Requirements

In the first six months of life, infants are dependent upon breast milk or an infant formula substitute for their nutrients. Infant growth is rapid and a continuous supply of nutrients is required. The infant's energy needs can be supplied by an average intake of 100-120 Kcal/Kg/day in the first four months, decreasing, as growth slows, to about 100 Kcal/Kg/day for the last six months of the first year. An infant should double birthweight at six months, and triple birthweight at one year.

One ounce (oz) of breast milk or substitute formula is about 20 Kcal/oz or 7 Kcal/100 mL. Infants begin consuming about 20 oz/day in Month 1 and progress to about 40 oz/day in Month 6. Water is important to infants and should supplement breast or formula feedings. A nursing mother must maintain a high intake of water (2-3 litres/day) to provide adequate dilution of her milk. She should avoid dehydration with diuretic substances, including alcoholic beverages (AB), teas, coffee, licorice, and herbal teas. Nursing mother's should take a well-balanced multivitamin-mineral supplement that includes Vitamin D, Calcium, iron, and zinc. The advice to mothers to drink extra cow's milk may be harmful to the infant who may develop milk protein allergy.

6.0.3 Food Allergy

One problem with mother's milk is that it may contain allergens which the mother has absorbed intact. Allergens derived from cow's milk may appear in the mother's milk and sensitize her child. The circuit of milk proteins through a mother's body, through the breast into the milk, into the infant's GIT, and into the infant's body is a remarkable biological fact! This free passage of food proteins through many body filters and defense systems demonstrates how porous we are to macromolecules.

Since food allergens from the mother's diet may appear in her breast milk, the lactating mother may have to modify her diet to protect her infant. Her restrictions may include the avoidance of milk products and other highly allergenic foods like eggs, peanuts, citrus fruits, chocolate, nuts, and, sometimes, cereal grains, certain meats, and fish. Breast-feeding mothers should avoid ingesting food and beverages with drug-like or toxic properties - alcoholic beverages, tea, coffee, chocolate, herbs, and spices.

Breast-feeding and smoking do not go together. Infant sensitization in utero and with breast feeding is not a simple matter, however, and even the most conscientious maternal avoidances will not assure complete protection against infant food allergy.

The effects of food antigens on an infant reflect a delicate and complex balance between tolerance and sensitivity. There are some apparent paradoxes involved. The infant who is fed large quantities of cow's milk will show tolerance to the acute effects of milk allergy - vomiting, abdominal pain, swelling, and shock - but, will manifest the more delayed results like eczema, colds, and diarrhea. The infant with little exposure will show less tolerance to the allergen and will react with the more dramatic acute responses, but may avoid the chronic delayed symptoms. Thus, the breast fed infant of a very careful mother has a greater risk of acute responses when allergenic foods are introduced than the casually fed infant with chronic symptoms. This is a distressing paradox, not confined to the infant immunological response, but observed in older children and adults as well.

Dr. John Gerrard, an authority on food allergy, reported this effect in his study of 19 children with IgE-mediated immediate reactions (IMD.E1) to milk, peanut, and/or egg.[16] He states:

> "Breast feeding is recommended because it provides optimal nutrition for most babies and, with placentally transferred antibody, protects the infant from a number of common infections: it also facilitates bonding between the mother and child. Breast feeding has also been said to protect the infant from the development of atopic diseases in general and eczema in particular. The degree of protection is not complete, for atopic diseases can develop in breast fed babies to foods ingested by the mother. It has been suggested that restricting the mother's intake of foods, such as cow's milk and egg will increase this protection; whereas increasing her intake of these and other foods will reduce this protection."

Dr. Gerrard's observations showed that the amount of a food eaten by the mother during pregnancy does not determine the sensitization of the infant - that acute allergic responses often occurred with the first ingestion of a food. If the mother is to significantly reduce food allergy in her infant, it appears that she must follow a rather vigorous hypoallergenic diet during her pregnancy and lactation. Half measures may reduce the infant risk, but do not eliminate it. If either of the parents have a history of infant food intolerances, vomiting, diarrhea, eczema, bronchitis, or asthma, the mother may consider it advisable to abstain from all dairy products, eggs, peanuts, and soya protein in an effort to minimize these potential problems in her infant.

The advice of a physician skilled in food allergy management is always desirable when preventive efforts are contemplated or infant feeding problems are encountered. Mother's nutrition can, and should, be supported by computed nutrient analysis and careful nutrient supplementation.

6.1 Introduction of Solid Foods

Infant feeding fashions change as we learn more about nutrition and food allergy. There is a concensus that solid foods may be a problem if introduced too early. In an adequately breast-fed infant, other foods are seldom required before five months and adequate nutrition can be readily maintained for six months. Iron, fluoride, and vitamin D may be supplemented in the mother's diet for the breast-fed infant. Cow's milk should probably be avoided during the first six months, although, in a pinch, boiled milk or formula made with condensed or evaporated milk may be acceptable. Commercial infant formulas are improvements over plain cow's milk and contain desirable amounts of added micronutrients, some of which are absent in cow's milk alone.

The infant bowel has matured sufficiently by five to six months for complex foods to be digested and absorbed with less risk of sensitization to antigenic food proteins. Infants of this age also should be able to sit with support, control head movements, and have adequate swallowing reflexes to ensure safe feeding. Solid foods may be slowly introduced and provide a critical transition from milk to other sources of nutrients.[17]

Premature introduction of solid foods has several risks:

1. Overfeeding with excessive weight gain and risk of life-long obesity.

2. Inadequate neuromuscular maturation, with problems swallowing, regurgitation, danger of aspiration and choking. Difficulty digesting

solid foods, with abdominal pain, diarrhea, gas, and risk of bowel surface damage.

3. Risk of inducing allergic responses to food. The infant has an immature GIT. From the allergy point of view, the infant GIT has limited defences against food proteins and other antigens, and is permeable to macromolecules. Absorption of large molecules from the bowel may trigger a variety of delayed allergic responses like eczema, bronchitis, or asthma, and may expose the infant to a high risk of immune-complex disease with serious target organ damage, and life-long food allergy.

The introduction of "solid" foods is begun slowly and gradually with soft or pureed foods. In a healthy, tolerant infant, new foods are best introduced one at a time at weekly intervals. One new food per week allows mother to detect both immediate and delayed adverse reactions to the new food and to discontinue it, if she is concerned. New foods are introduced by teaspoon quantity, and the serving size is progressively increased, as the infant becomes accustomed to the new food.

Hypersensitive infants may not tolerate many foods or such a fast pace of introduction. A few foods from the Phase 1 Core Diet list may be all an infant can handle during the first year. Nutritional support with a hypoallergenic formula or ENF may be required if the infant cannot breast feed for any reason.

A variety of food introduction schedules have been suggested. Infant cereals mixed with milk are the usual North American practice. A rice cereal (with iron added) has some advantages over wheat-based cereals. Gluten allergy or intolerance is common in the food-sensitive child, and wheat products are avoided at first. Oats and barley may be the best tolerated cereal grains, but their acceptibility is not assumed (all 4 cereal grains - wheat, rye, oats, and barley are excluded on the Core Diet). Pureed vegetables should be introduced before fruits. Egg white (albumin) and nuts are avoided in the first year.

Phase 1 Core Diet foods are the best first foods in approximately the following order:

Rice cereal	Yams	Squash
Pears	Turkey	Chicken
Carrots	Green Beans	Rice
Peas	Broccoli	Rice cakes
Peaches	Zucchini	

All foods are well-cooked and pureed at first. New foods are best introduced one at a time at weekly intervals. To prepare infant food at home, steam cook it and puree it with an infant food press or a blender. A blender is a very useful, relatively inexpensive kitchen tool which can transform fruit and steam-cooked vegetables into purees, creamy soups, and, with the addition of more water, juices. Homemade juices, from vegetables and fruit, are better tolerated than store-bought products.

Commercially prepared foods are suitable. I have been favorably impressed by the educational efforts of the Heinz and Gerber companies in promoting appropriate infant feeding practices. The Heinz recommendations fully recognize the problems of food allergy and recommend a food introduction schedule which minimizes the risk of food allergy. They include charts of food compositions and reassurances that their products do not contain salt, sugar, nor additives. Gerber "First Foods" are single foods cooked and pureed without additives. Infant and Junior foods make a mother's work easier and can be recommended, despite our general ban on packaged and bottled food. Canned peaches and pears, packed in their own juice rather than in sugar syrup, can also be recommended.

Vitamin A 1500 IU and D 200 IU, Iron 10 mg and Fluoride 100 mcg can be given as an infant supplement during the first six months.

On the Core Diet we avoid foods that contain milk, wheat, gluten, egg white, albumin, whey, casein, and hydrolysed proteins.

By nine months the food mixtures can contain some lumps to encourage chewing. By the end of the first year foods can be well-cooked and cut in small manageable pieces at the table. Infants completing their first year are capable of feeding themselves and show distinct food preferences. The gradual introduction of a full complement of adult foods is desirable. The biggest favor that parents can do for their child's long-term well being is to develop the vegetable habit. Approximately two thirds of a child's total calories should come from mixed vegetables and grains, with rice being the favorite. Some fish should be included in their diet, if tolerated, after the first year. I disagree with recommendations to include 25% dairy products and believe this recommendation should be 0-10%. Yogurt is the preferred milk-food.

Milk should be quickly eliminated from the diets of symptomatic children, since allergy to milk is the great imitator of diverse diseases.

Some infants are really stubborn and new food introduction is a slow process. Often infants reject a novel smell or flavor; the new food may have to mixed in very small quantities into a previously accepted food and the amount slowly increased. Strong aversions to a new food, appearing days to weeks after its introduction, probably mean an adverse reaction and feeding of the food should be discontinued for several weeks. Mother should keep a record of these incidents. The infant cannot tell you that his throat is sore, that he has heartburn, a headache, or abdominal pain; he can only avoid or reject the food linked to his symptoms. He does not think about this connection; the avoidance or aversion is a conditioned, reflexive response. Vomiting is the most dramatic form of food rejection and is always decided by a machine-level program in the brain stem, which responds to chemosensory input from the nose, mouth, and throat. Once a conditioned reflex is established, the sight, smell, or taste of food can trigger aversive behavior, including vomiting. Conscious decisions have nothing to do with it and the infant is not "attention-seeking"; he is suffering and needs help.

Phase 2 foods can be introduced after month 10 -12 at a pace which suits the child's interest and tolerance. Food intake tends to drop in the second year. Infants triple their birthweight in the first year and have a huge appetite. The rate of growth declines during the second year, and so may the child's appetite. It is common for 1-3 year old infants to refuse foods and to cycle through single food preferences for weeks at a time. Mothers may worry about reduced food intake and attempt forced feeding - this is always a mistake.

Too much sugar intake as cookies, candies, or fruit and fruit juice may spoil the child's appetite for vegetable foods, for example. Reduce the child's sugar intake and fruit portions in favor of increased vegetable portions. The Core Diet proportioning rules are an excellent guide to feeding all children even when major diet revision is not required.

Fussy and picky eating along with physical symptoms means food problems until proven otherwise. Children with food allergy typically become eating specialists - compulsively eating a small number of "favorite" foods and refusing the rest. Some food aversions are protective - the food may cause symptoms. Other food aversion is compulsive or addictive and may signal the presence of food allergy. Vegetable foods are the first foods refused by 1-3 year olds with food allergy, often in favor of compulsive eating of fruit juices, dairy or wheat products. It is important to recognize and correct abnormal food-body interactions at this time.

6.2 Feeding Older Children

Children and adolescents are among our most vulnerable citizens. They depend on their parents, school and culture to guide them toward healthy, sane living. Their food supply tends to be the most synthetic of any age group. Food manufacturers and vendors advertise their synthetic, processed foods directly to youngsters, and generally succeed in marketing their products. The result is that children and adolescents ingest a large amount of inappropriate molecular nonsense. Their health and sanity is at risk.

6.2.1 Nutrient Deficiencies

Concern for nutritional deficiencies in children has led to routine vitamin supplementation of staple foods- bread, breakfast cereals, and fruit juices. Vitamins D and C are often obtained as food supplements. Further concern for nutritional deficiencies in children of poor families in the U.S. inspired nationwide food assistance programs. Preschool children have been given supplemental foods with measureable improvement in nutrient intake. Poverty obviously limits food choices and availability, leading to malnutrition. Despite supplemental feedings and improvement in nutritional status of children of poor black families in Memphis;[18] 18% were deficient in Vitamin A, 13 % were deficient in vitamin C, 18 % in riboflavin, and 17% in iron. Overall concern for iron deficiency in children led to the widely debated recommendation to supplement flour with iron. Iron has been added to infant cereals to cover the deficient period from six months onward.

Children of more affluent families may also suffer malnutrition in the form of caloric excess, and nutrient disproportion - "Affluent MalNutrition", or AMN for short. Food choices tend to be limited to the three new food groups - fast frozen or take-out. Children tend to avoid eating vegetable foods, and seldom achieve balanced diets by eating primary or "natural" foods. Their high intake of commercially processed, manufactured foods exposes them to high fat, sugar and salt intakes, and to a bewildering number of food additives and contaminants.

Standard food rules suggest that children eat milk, eggs, meat, and whole grain cereals as staple foods. Is this good advice? Official food selection advice probably misdirects 30-40% of children into illness patterns caused by food allergy to these staple foods. Boxed cereal and milk is the most common breakfast. The cereal has been nutritionally fortified, and so has the milk; nutrient intake may be marginally satisfactory, but what is the impact of the food on the child as a whole? A peanut butter-jam sandwich and a carton of milk (PBJS&M) must be the most common school lunch, followed by the most common afternoon symptoms - flushing, fatigue, irritability, and inability to concentrate. Nutrient analysis of the PBJS&M lunch may not be all that bad, but the whole body physiological effects of the food tend to be a problem, at least for a significant subpopulation of children. Allergy to milk, wheat, and peanuts lead the list of problems attached to the PBJS&M lunch.

Television is an important determinant of food preferences through the food advertising directed at children. Watching TV also keeps children physically idle, and snacking on junk foods. Drs. Dietz and Gortmaker[19] reported that for each additional TV hour per day, the rate of obesity increased by 1 to 3%. They state:

> "Watching television requires no energy in excess of resting metabolic rates, and may reduce the time spent in more energy-expensive activities. The foods heavily advertised on children's television, and more likely to be consumed by children watching increased amounts of television are calorically dense foods such as sugared breakfast cereals, candy bars, cakes, cookies, and carbonated beverages...the prevalence of obesity could be reduced, and the disease could in some cases be prevented by a reduction in television viewing and an increase in other activities."

The three principal hazards of TV are then:

1. Videocy
2. Obesity & AMN
3. Atrophy (of bones, muscle, energy and creativity)

Children of well-motivated parents tend to receive routine vitamin supplements. In an Ontario study,[20] 90% of children were given multisupplements at some time; 34% of children received regular supplements, and another 37% were given supplements in the winter. Parents often use vitamins as first line "drugs" to treat colds, fatigue, or ill-defined symptoms. Vitamin overdose in young children is a problem, especially with the flavored, sugared chewable brands. The risk of overdose to children increases with the number of multiple supplements in the home; from 1.5% for one supplement to 8% for 4 supplements per child-year.

Despite supplementation, some nutrients remain in short supply in childrens' diets. In one study,[21] folic acid and pyridoxine (B6) were in short supply. Studies of populations overall do not tell us about individual children. Children tend to become food specialists and idiosyncratic eaters. I have found great variation in nutrient content of children's diets, and routinely find nutrient deficiencies. The general advice that "no supplements are needed, given a normal well-balanced diet"; hardly applies to the real world. Many children suffer from nutrient disproportion, and need diet revision, followed by computed nutrient analysis. Nutrient deficiencies may include vitamin D, pyridoxine, folic acid, calcium, potassium, fluoride, and iron, and are corrected by supplementation. "Childrens' vitamins" may not be correctly formulated, and often have inferior ingredients, with sugars, dyes, and fillers - all may cause allergic reactions. Ideally, an individually prescribed supplementation program should follow a computed nutrient analysis of the child's actual diet. Laboratory measurements may be required to assess the absorption and utilization of nutrients in children who are not doing well.

6.2.2 Adolescents

Teenagers have notoriously poor diets. Among the many adjustment upheavals that teenagers experience, changes in food preferences, junk-food socialization, alcoholic beverages, and drug use all conspire against the health and mental well-being of adolescents. Nutrient disproportion, and deficiencies are common and difficult to correct, because of teenagers resistance to rational approaches to their existence. Food allergy is common in this age group and almost never correctly diagnosed.

Teenagers tend to assume they can eat and drink as they please without negative consequences and practice body neglect, while aspiring to have perfect bodies. Their many health problems are often diet-related, and they need special consideration before they develop workable insights into self-management. Eating disorders develop readily in teenage girls who are caught between compulsive eating cycles, and a desire for an attractive body. Nutrient deficiencies and addictive patterns of eating maintain the abberrant food intake. Casual vitamin-mineral supplementation alone does not correct seriously-flawed food selection.

In our experience, teenagers between the ages of 15 and 20 are the "lost generation". Many are sick and depressed from wrong food intake, but very few will admit their symptoms, and fewer will comply with the Core Diet instructions. Even well-motivated teenagers who are seriously ill, with supportive, loving families have trouble staying with a safe hypoallergenic diet. Their propensity to "hang-out" in restaurants, and to seek immediate gratification usually cancels the Core Diet instructions. We all share food and drink in rituals of membership in social groups and teenagers have a special need for peer group approval.

Parents should do everything in their power to encourage healthy diet revision in a teenager who is ill or emotionally disturbed. Following the Core Diet is very difficult. Not following the Core Diet may be catastrophic. Food control is the first positive step toward healthy self-determination. Positive food choices promise positive life choices and usually means that the teenager will also avoid abusing alcohol and drugs.

Glossary	
AA	Amino Acid
BUN	Blood Urea Nitrogen
CHO	Carbohydrate
CCHO	Complex Carbohydrate
DF	Derivative Foods
EPA	Eicosapentanenoic Acid
FA	Fatty Acid
GIT	Gastro-intestinal Tract
MALT	Mucosa Associated Lymphatic Tissue
MSG	Monosodium Glutamate
NH3	Ammonia
NP	Nutritional Programming
PC	Phosphatidyl Choline
PCB's	Polychlorinated Biphenyls
PF	Primary Foods
PUFA	Poly Unsaturated Fatty Acids
RDA	Recommended Daily Allowance
TCCD	Tetrachlorodebenzo-para Dioxin

Chapter 7

NUTRITIONAL SCIENCE REVISITED

This chapter is a mini-course on basic nutrition. If you find some of this text difficult to read, do not give up. As your involvement with food intensifies, questions come up, or friend's opinions need to be considered - use the text as reference material. More detailed, technical treatment of this subject is found in "Nutritional Programming" the reference text for the Core Diet series. References to "NP" indicate nutritional programming concepts, and new a different way to approach diet design. The Core Diet can be thought of as a Nutritional Program, designed to resolve current illness, improve nutritional status generally, and prevent endemic disease in the longer Term.

7.1 Basic Concepts of Nutrition

7.1.1 Primary and Derivative Foods

We can recognize two kinds of foods: Primary (PF) and Derivative (DF). Primary foods are in their close-to-natural state, and come directly from the farm or the sea. Both fresh or frozen plant or animal tissues can be considered PF, as long as they are not processed in any way. The optimal food is unsprayed, garden-fresh produce from rich healthy organic soils, free of acid rain, radioactive isotopes, and other forms of air pollution. All foods which are preserved, processed, manufactured, cooked, baked, smoked, packaged, or bottled are derivatives. Derivative foods, of course, have increased burdens of non-nutrient chemicals - additives and contaminants.

7.1.2 Nutrients Redefined

What are nutrients? There are forty simple substances considered essential nutrients. No food is nourishing until it has been carefully and completely digested into individual nutrients. Nutrients must then be absorbed, processed in the liver, and passed on to our cells' metabolic machinery. Protein should not be considered a "nutrient". The meaning of a protein molecule is totally different from the meaning of the amino acids which make it up, just as these words have meaning which their letters alone do not imply. Fat is not a nutrient. Only some carbohydrates are nutrients.

7.1.3 Class A-1 Molecules: Essential Nutrients

1. *Macronutrients:* These are the bulk supply to the body consisting of sugars, fatty acids, and amino acids. These molecules must be supplied in sufficient quantity to fuel the body and to replace structural material lost through secretion, excretion, or injury. Minerals, required in milligram to gram quantity (calcium, magnesium, sodium, and potassium), may also be considered macronutrients. There are essential and non-essential macronutrients in our food supply.

2. *Micronutrients:* These are the essential vitamins and minerals, required in small amounts as co-factors or catalysts to enzymes. Enzymes are responsible for the millions of different molecular transactions which sustain our life. Many enzymes must have one or two vitamins and at least one critical mineral co-factor to function.

The basic idea of life chemistry has the following form:

Nutrients------> Enzyme + Vitamin + Mineral----> Cell Product

For example, to make the neurotransmitter, serotonin, you need the amino acid, tryptophan, as the raw material. Once tryptophan arrives at the appropriate place inside a neuron in your brain, a molecular workshop containing two enzymes and the vitamin, VM.B6, transforms tryptophan to serotonin. Serotonin is then transferred to the sending end of the neuron (the terminal bouton of the axon) where it is used as a molecular messenger to carry information across the synapse to the receiving neuron.

The serotonin synthesis equation is:

Step 1. Tryptophan----> 5-Hydroxytrytophan

Step 2. 5-Hydroxytryptophan (5HT)---->Serotonin
via enzyme 5HT-Decarboxylase

7.1.4 Class A Molecules: Four Groups

Let us define nutrients as Class A Molecules. Nutrients have specific destinations in cells and often display normal, regular, predictable habits once inside a body. Class A molecules tend to make sense to body and brain cells, although there is no guarantee that a population of class A molecules will make sense in all circumstances. Many so-called "nutrients" are not essential in our diets since, given a normal and proper metabolism, most of our molecular needs can be synthesized with an adequate supply of the essential nutrients.

There are several substances which may be considered "Accessory" nutrients, like choline, biotin, EPA, gamma-linoleic acid, carnitine, taurine, and tyrosine. While these molecules can be synthesized within, they may be needed in the food supply when production is deficient or utilization is blocked. There are specific inborn errors of metabolism which require accessory nutrients to be present in or added to the diet.

7.1.5 Essential Nutrients: A1

When nutritional theorists fail to make the distinction between true nutrients and the prenutrient food substances from which we derive nutrients, confusion arises. The classification proposed here tries to resolve this confusion. Class A molecules are divided into four subgroups:

Class A-1 are the *Essential Nutrients*. There are about 40 essential nutrients in this class.

Class A-2 are *Prenutrients*, the larger molecules common to all foods which yield the essential nutrients after digestion has dissembled these larger molecules into smaller ones. A2's are usually classified as carbohydrates, fats, and proteins.

Class A-3 are the non-essential or *Optional Nutrients*. These molecules are used normally in cellular metabolism, but are not missed if they are absent. The sugar galactose; the fatty acids oleic, stearic caproic, or caprylic; the amino acids alanine, aspartic, cystine, proline, and serine are all examples of A-3 molecules. These substances are all metabolically significant. Some of them may make important contributions to our well-being which we do not always appreciate. Other A-3's may be problems for some people with specific metabolic intolerances, and can be removed from the diet with benefits, but no apparent adverse effects.

Class A-4 are *Accessory Nutrients*. These substances may be considered for inclusion in the A-1 list, if more information supports their benefits, or special needs are demonstrated for some individuals. The amino acid, L-carnitine, is an A-3 molecule, produced in our cells; on occasion, we can consider it as an A-4 or even A-1 substance. The indications for carnitine use are found in subsequent chapters. Choline is definitely an A-4, as are EPA and GLA. Inositol and bioflavinoids are doubtful candidates.

A1 Molecules or Essential nutrients

Amino Acids	Elements	Vitamins
Isoleucine	Calcium	Ascorbic Acid
Leucine	Chloride	Vitamin A
Lysine	Copper	Folic Acid
Methionine	Iodine	Niacin
Phenylalanine	Iron	Pyridoxine
Thryonine	Magnesium	Riboflavin
Tryptophan	Manganese	Thiamin
Valine	Phosphorus	Vitamin B12
	Potassium	Vitamins D
	Sodium	Vitamin E
	Zinc	Vitamin K
FA: Linoleic acid.		

A3 Optional Group

Arginine	Fluoride	Biotin
Histidine	Molybdenum	Pantothenic acid
Linolenic A.	Selenium	

A4: Accessory Nutrients
Choline, Silicon, Lithium?
EPA, Gamma–Linoleic acid
Tyrosine, Taurine, L–carnitine, L–Ornithine

Silicon is not usually considered essential for human nutrition, but is essential for many animals. Silicon compounds probably should be treated as A-4 substances, ready for inclusion in the A-1 list, especially when ENFormulas are designed or restricted diets limit access to silicon compounds. Other candidates for accessory nutrient status include inositol, bioflavinoids, and the non-essential fatty acids, gamma-linoleic acid and eicosapentanenoic acid (EPA). Occasionally, false candidates for nutrient status are popularized by the new alchemist subculture. Pangamic acid or "Vitamin B15" is an example of a proposed, but unlikely A4 substance, which will never become A1. Pangamic acid has proved not to be a discrete substance and may be more toxic than helpful.

7.2 A2: Prenutrients: Carbohydrate, Fat, Protein

The A2 level description is the first level approximation of the biological action of food. The concept of molecular size and identity becomes very important to us when we consider the problem of food allergy. Proteins are large molecules, containing hundreds of amino acids. We do not utilize protein to make protein. We dismantle the protein into little pieces, amino acids, bring those inside, transport them to all cells, who then use them to construct new proteins. The building up of large molecules by plants (photosynthesis) and the breaking down of the same large molecules by animals is the basis of life on earth. The sun energizes the whole cycle and our metabolic energy is indirectly an expression of the sun's energy. One can make an excellent case for staying close to the sun in choosing proper foods. Staying close to the sun means eating plant tissues. This is also thought of as the "top" of the food chain, the most biologically efficient location for a food consumer.

The idea that we should eat food combinations that result in a definitive proportion of fat, CHO, and protein is basic to nutritional thinking. Standard recommendation suggests the proportions:

CARBOHYDRATE....53%
FAT.............35%
PROTEIN.........12%

The main area of dispute in this recommendation is the proportion of fat and carbohydrate. Recently increased concern about the role of dietary fat, especially animal fat, in arterial disease and cancer has prompted suggestions that the fat proportion be decreased and complex carbohydrate increased. NP favors increased vegetable content of the diet and suggests the following proportions:

CARBOHYDRATE.....68%
FAT..............20%
PROTEIN..........12%

The short-form notation for CFP proportions is C68:F20:P12.

7.2.1 Food Group Proportion

The idea of A2 proportion is linked to food group choices. Standard nutritional advice encourages us to choose foods from four food groups:

	Daily Servings
Grains	*3*
Dairy	*2*
Vegetables and Fruit	*2*
Meat or Alternative	*2*

The food-group proportion rules and the daily servings make diet design a relatively simple undertaking. Dieticians use these rules in recommending "normal diets". Medically-altered diets have tended to follow the same basic rules, simply altering proportions. Diverse weight reduction diets have altered the proportion rules in every conceivable way, without any scheme demonstrating weight-reduction superiority.

The proportion rules are programming precepts. Obviously, the rules are too general to be all that useful. We would like to know more about the different kinds of fats, carbohydrates and proteins. The distinction between saturated fat, found in animal foods, and polyunsaturated fats, found in vegetable oils, is important. The distinction between sugar carbohydrate and complex vegetable carbohydrate is similarly important. The food group idea has one major limitation. It is not applicable to everyone. Many people suffer adverse reactions to food or have other reasons for not eating from one or other of the food groups.

The Core Diet is programmed to reduce the negative consequences of eating allergenic and otherwise problematic foods. The exclusion of foods from major groups - dairy, cereal grains, eggs, and citrus fruits - is based on the higher frequency of adverse reactions to these foods. The Core Diet is specific about food choices, and sets goals for amounts and timing of eating. Your task is to custom fit the food choices to your child's needs. The Core Diet begins with the following food allotments. As you add foods, you adjust the portion sizes to your child's needs and tolerances. You will re-write this list after 4 weeks and again in 8-10 weeks as you more fully define the best choices on the Core Diet.)

7.2.2 Food Groups and Portions Per Day:

Cereal Grains & Flour	[0]	Rice	[3]
Grain Alternates	[1]	Beverages (all)	[0]
Dairy Group	[0]	Eggs	[0]
Green Vegetables	[2]	Other Vegetables	[3]
Citrus Fruits	[0]	Other Fruits	[2]
Soya Products	[1]	Nuts	[0]
Meats (mammalian)	[0]	Poultry	[2]
Fish	[0]	Other Seafood	[0]
Vitamin suppl.	[2]	Mineral Suppl.	[2]

The sample program includes an instruction to take vitamin and mineral supplements, since some nutrient shortages are likely with the limited food choices in the early stages of diet revision.

7.3 Carbohydrates

Carbohydrates (CHO) are sugar-base molecules of great diversity. Complex carbohydrates (CCHO), like starch, are found in plant foods everywhere. Starch is a polymer or long string of sugar molecules, just as a protein is a long string of amino acids. Starch-containing plants are the universal staple foods. The success of the core diet depends on increasing vegatable carbohydrate to about 2/3's of daily caloric requirements.

Rice, millet, potato, and maize have long been the major carbohydrate-supplying food plants, and more recently the cereal grains and their flours have dominated as staples, especially in the industrial nations. Currently rice, wheat, and maize or corn are the world's most important staple foods. The American diet has become an eclectic melange of foods. Most of us have traded the sense of a traditional staple diet for an improvised, often whimsical, sometimes careless selection of foods. What should eat tonight? Let's go to the new Greek restaurant...I want Chinese food...no, let's have a pizza...In the rest of the world, food shortage is more of a problem, and people in third world countries rely on a single staple plant for 50-90% of their daily calories.

Vegetables are a major source of complex carbohydrates. In the US about 15% of agricultural production is devoted to vegetable cultivation. High-starch vegetables tend to be roots or tubers like potatoes, yams, turnips, winter squashes, carrots, and beets. Yam is an important staple of tropical climates. The green leafy vegetables are more chemically diverse and interesting foods, supplying less digestable carbohydrate, but more vitamins, minerals, and non-digestible fiber. Legumes are important vegetables, since they are high in protein, fatty acids, and are almost universally available. We eat seeds of 30 or so common legume species. Soybeans are perhaps the most important legume, supplying carbohydrate as well as oil, and protein. Beans, peas, lentils, and peanuts are the other common legumes.

One of the fallacies of popular nutrition is the belief that food remains constant. We tend to assume a great deal about the sameness of things, which are really constantly changing. Among plant crops there is remarkable diversity. Potatoes, for example, are lumped together as the same food. Biochemical analysis of potatoes, however, reveals remarkable diversity. Every variety of European potato has a unique set of proteins. This diversity would completely foil efforts to standardize therapeutic diets if we were not aware of it.

7.3.1 Sugar

Sugar is a well discussed, often maligned, and greatly misunderstood food component. The only true nutrient sugars are glucose, and fructose. These are the simplest CHO molecules, known by their single ring structure as monosaccharides. Glucose is the fuel of all living things, supplying energy to all living cells, plant and animal. The creation of glucose begins in plants with the magic of photosynthesis. The sun's photons are the original energy source used by the chloroplasts of leaves to drive carbon, hydrogen, and oxygen atoms together to form glucose. Plants then use the newly synthesized glucose to fuel all their other synthetic processes, constructing tissues so that animals have food to eat. Fructose, common in fruits, is the first cousin of glucose.

Sucrose is the sugar that is commonly called "sugar", often with pejorative connotations. Sucrose Is the dominant sugar in most of our sweeteners, and appears in refined form as white table sugar. Brown sugars, and molasses are cruder sugar products which contain the same sucrose, in the presence of many other substances, not yet removed. The preference for brown sugars, syrups, molasses, and honey, in place of reflned white sugar is not based on any important biological information. White table sugar has the advantage of containing less extraneous molecules, and contaminants. Honey is preferable only by taste and implication (visions of bees, flowers, summer days...), but contains the same sugars, glucose and fructose. Honey also contains bees' wings, legs, poop, pollens, and other assorted hive contaminants, and may offer some allergic reactions to microsensitive individuals. Honey also carries the spores of the botulinus bacteria, and should not be fed to infants, since the spores can germinate in their intestine producing the deadly botulinus toxin. I personally prefer honey by taste, implication, and a lingering identification with Winnie the Pooh.

7.3.2 Carbohydrate Chemistry: Saccharides

The basic sugars, glucose, fructose, galactose, mannose, are the building blocks of larger more complex carbohydrates. These "monosaccharides" contain 6 carbon atoms, and typically form a six-sided ring structure. The energy density of sugars is 4 kcal/gm. Lactate or lactic acid is the 3-carbon fragment of these sugars, produced as the sugar is oxidized as fuel. The same sugar has two mirror-image forms, determined by the rotation of a test light beam through its crystal in the laboratory. Biologically active sugars are the "D" form, rotating light to the "dextro" or right side. D-Glucose is referred to as "dextrose". The general formula for a 6-C ring sugar, or hexose is:

$$C6.H12.O6$$

A group of 5-carbon sugars, pentoses, are also important. Arabinose, Ribose, and Xylose are the most common pentoses. Ribose has its starring role in genetic material, formed into ribonucleic acid, which gives RNA and DNA their long names. Polymers of arabinose are gums like araban. The fate of ingested pentoses is not well known, and remains one of the holes in the knowledge of food-body interaction.

Sugar alcohols are first cousins of the basic monosaccharides. A simple chemical exchange, adding a hydrogen ion or proton to a sugar's double bonded oxygen, $C = O$, produces a sugar alcohol with a C-OH group. Sorbitol is such a beast, found as a food additive. Sorbitol is GRAS (Generally Recognized As Safe). Most ingested sorbitol is not absorbed, but passes onto the colon, where bacteria turn it into hydrogen gas. Absorbed sorbitol is metabolized to fructose. Mannitol is another C-OH sweetener, added to commercial foods. Inositol is another sugar alcohol of questionable status. Mice and rats seem to require it in their diets, but we apparently do not. Inositol may considered a candidate for accessory nutrient status for use in selected individuals, although the criteria for selection are currently unknown. Inositol is combined with 6 phosphate groups in cereal grains to form phytic acid, a undesirable substance, which binds minerals and prevents their absorption.

The next group of common sugars consists of two basic sugars, and are therefore called "Disaccharides". Lactose is the sugar in breast and cow's milk, and contains glucose and galactose. Sucrose, as discussed above, is glucose and fructose. Maltose is glucose and glucose.

7.3.3 Carbohydrate Polymers: Polysaccharides

Large Carbohydrate molecules form the structure of plants, and to a lesser extent, animals. A carbohydrate polymer, or polysaccharide, is a string of sugar molecules linked together. The cell walls of plants are constructed of elaborate polysaccharides made from 12 basic sugars. Cellulose is the main structural carbohydrate, and is a polymer of glucose units, linked together to form a fiber. We lack digestive enzymes to break down cellulose, and therefore miss some of the nutritive value of plants. Vegetarian ruminants, like cows, utilize special stomachs, which host bacterial populations that break down cellulose.

Starch is the most obvious, and most valuable polysaccharide. The starch molecule is tree-like, with branches of varying length. Starch digestion begins in the mouth with salivary amylase, and continues in the small intestine with pancreatic amylase. Short chains of glucoses are referred to as alpha-dextrin, maltotriose (3GL), and maltose (2GL). Glucoamylase breaks these short chains down to individual glucose molecules which are absorbed. Starch is probably our best fuel, supplying sustained release glucose. For many years "starchy foods" were maligned by dietary advice, especially weight loss advice. Fortunately, the trend has reversed, and now "complex carbohydrates" (CCHO) are recommended highly. The only important CCHO which can be digested to supply nutrient sugar is starch. Other CCHO's tend to be undigestible and form the fiber content of the diet.

There are several different types of carbohydrate polymer in fruit and vegetables that we are unable to digest. This material passes through the GIT as ruffage or fiber, undergoing modification, and digestion by colon micro-organisms. Several fibers have benevolent roles. The benefit seems to be the absorption or neutralization of the irritation or toxicity of other foods. Carbohydrate fiber contributes to the well-hydrated bulk of soft, easily-passed stools. Increased dietary fiber over a life-time is associated with decreased incidence of bowel cancer, and cardiovascular disease.

7.4 Proteins and Amino Acids

Food supplies the building materials to permit continuous cellular renewal and growth. Protein forms a major part of our structure. Most of our body protein is recycled and we do well by ingesting very little protein. About 3% of the total body protein is recycled everyday (approximately 200 grams worth). In a healthy child net protein loss in a day may be as low as 1-2 grams. Dietary requirements for protein increase with activity growth, and with protein losses, especially following injury or during illness.

The average American diet supplies 11-14% of total calories as protein, or 25-100 gms/day in children under 16. Protein digestion and absorption are generally efficient. A minimum average protein intake is approximately 25-30 grams for a normal child. Since all amino acids contain a nitrogen atom (N), protein balance is synonymous with nitrogen balance. When nitrogen intake exceeds nitrogen loss, there is net protein synthesis. Anabolism, or tissue construction, prevails. When nitrogen losses exceed intake, protein tissue is being broken down and catabolism prevails. A major problem of malnutrition, following surgery, injury, or illness, is catabolism of tissues with protein wasting. Adequate intake of energy molecules, both carbohydrate and fats, are said to "spare protein," permitting a small protein intake to maintain positive nitrogen balance. In metabolic studies, the total amount of nitrogen intake is compared with the total excretion of nitrogen to assess protein balance.

7.4.1 Ammonia is Protein Exhaust

Excess amino acids may be converted to fuel. When amino acids are "burned" as a fuel, ammonia (NH_3) is the waste product. Ammonia must be carried to the liver, converted to UREA and excreted by the kidneys. One of the penalties of amino acid excess is ammonia excess, a potential cause of body malfunction following a high protein meal. The blood measurement of urea nitrogen (BUN) shows the net balance between urea production by the liver and excretion by the kidneys. The BUN rises in kidney failure and serves as measure of ammonia or nitrogen toxicity. In liver disease, reduced ability to synthesize urea leads to ammonia accumulation.

Ammonia is neurotoxic and contributes to the syndrome of brain dysfunction in liver failure - hepatic encephalopathy. All patients with reduced kidney or liver function are required to restrict protein, since their ability to handle the nitrogen waste of oxidized amino acids is limited. Fluctating levels of ammonia in "normal" children is one systemic variable that influences brain cell function, and must be consider whenever brain function is abnormal. Some children are born with metabolic abnormalities in the handling of amino acids and ammonia - they often present with malfunctioning brains. The proper study of these children includes blood and urine ammonia and amino acid measurements with and without protein or amino acid loading. Amino acid tolearance tests are not yet clinical routines in diagnosing children's behavioral problems but soon should be.

7.4.2 Essential and Non-Essential

Amino acids are the alphabet characters of body proteins. Proteins are chains of amino acids linked together like beads on a necklace. The individual amino acids fall into two groups; the essential AA's, which must be ingested, and the non-essential AA's, which can be synthesized in the body and need not appear in the food. Nine amino acids are considered essential, while another 11 or so can be synthesized from the essential amino acids. This is a rule of thumb only. Essential amino acids may not always be required continuously and non-essential amino acids may become quite essential for normal functioning, when metabolic defects block synthesis of them.

There are other amino acids which appear in nature and are not included in protein structure. These odd amino acids appear especially in plants, where they may have roles as insect deterrents. An occasional non-nutrient amino acid may be useful in the food supply as an accessory nutrient - taurine is a prime candidate.

Essential Amino Acids
Histidine	Isoleucine
Leucine	Lysine
Methionine	Phenylalanine
Threonine	Tryptophan
Valine	

Nonessential Amino Acids
Alanine	Arginine
Aspartic Acid	Cystine
Glutamic Acid	Glycine
Proline	Serine
Tyrosine	

Accessory Nutrient Amino Acids
Taurine	L-carnitine	L-Ornithine

7.4.3 Amino Acids: Requirements & Intolerances

Amino acids appear to be relatively easy to obtain in adequate amounts, even on simple vegetarian diets with no meat, fish, eggs, or milk, provided that different vegetables are combined. Mixing a legume with a grain or with a tuber should provide a complete amino acid mixture, as well as a good variety of vitamins and minerals Some of the non-essential AA's may become essential if their synthesis is blocked by enzyme deficiencies. In order for protein synthesis to proceed, all the amino acids must be supplied at the same time. The highest "quality" protein contains all the essential amino acids. Proteins of animal origin are high quality. Since we are mammals, we can expect other mammalian proteins to have similar amino acid combinations. Plant proteins may be very different in their composition compared to our own. Plant proteins often are deficient in lysine, threonine, and tryptophan. Vegetables can be combined to achieve the complete essential amino acid repertoire. Corn or maize, for example, is deficient in lysine (and high in leucine) - people dependent on it as a staple food suffer "protein malnutrition" because of the missing amino acid. Many years of corn-breeding research have produced hybrid corns, with increased total protein and increased lysine content in particular. The substitution of the newer corn hybrids may eliminate protein malnutrition among corn-dependent populations.

Patients on limited diets seem may do better than predicted - they somehow conserve essential amino acids, synthesize them de novo, or obtain them from non-ingested sources. Synthesis of essential amino acids may occur in the colon, by colonic bacteria.[22]. Diets low in protein but high in non-digestible carbohydrates (plant materials), and low in fat sustain most of the earth's people and may represent an optimal mix. Often, a minimal diet with marginally adequate nutrient intake will improve, not degrade, health. A minimal diet presents minimal problems and nonsense programs to one's metabolism. A protein deficient diet, in other words, may be better tolerated than a protein excess diet.

Some laboratories offer blood and urine amino acid profiles, as evidence of normal or abnormal amino acid metabolism. We would like to know all the details of amino acid processing inside of body cells, especially the brain. Amino acids in the brain likely decide much about our mental life. Whenever questions arise about hidden amino acid abnormalities, we are frustrated by lack of data. Simple empirical tests - trials of single amino acid ingestion - are immediately available, practical, and relatively safe, although major discomforts, and troubling disturbances in brain function can be expected. The clinical strategy of nutritional programming is to alter food intake and adjust nutrient proportions until good results are obtained. If the NP directives are intelligent and heuristics are in place, empirical regulation of metabolism works well enough to be immediately practical. The development of better measuring and interpretation tools has the highest priority, especially in the diagnosing and treatment of brain dysfunctional diseases like childhood autism and adult schizophrenia.

The patterns of the major inborn errors of metabolism have minor versions in individuals who are less obviously dysfunctional. The major amino acid disorders are readily diagnosed by clinical and laboratory examinations; the minor manifestations are difficult to detect.

7.5 Fat and Cholesterol

Dietary fats are a heterogeneous mixture consisting of about 93 percent triglycerides, six percent phospholipids and lesser amounts of sphingomyelins, glycolipids, cholesterol and phytosterols. Fat is usually fully digested, with less than five percent remaining unabsorbed, and excreted in the feces. If fat digestion is impaired, by pancreatic enzyme deficiency, an oily diarrhea results, with foamy, floating stools (steatorrhea). Ingested fat mostly consists of triglycerides. The molecule, glycerol, acts like a rack to which 3 fatty acids (FA) attach. There are many different fatty acids, and their individual metabolic effects are not well known.

7.5.1 Fatty Acid Chemistry

FA are chains of carbon molecules with the form, -C-C-C-. If carbon atoms are joined by two of their available four bonds, -C=C=C-, the FA is described as "polyunsaturated" (PUFA), a single bond, -C-C-C- is saturated. The double bond facilitates molecular re-arrangement in the body, and everyone has been told that -C=C=C- is better than -C-C-C-. There is, however, evidence that increased total fat is harmful, regardless of the bonding arrangements. Increased incidence of skin, breast, and colon cancer may be correlated with increased intake of PUFA. The exact nature of each fatty acids may be more of a specific determinant than its general biochemical properties. There is a scarcity of knowledge about the specific roles of individual FA.

Vegetable oils, liquid at room temperature, tend to be unstaturated, and animal fats, solid at room temperature tend to be saturated. Margarines are made from vegetable oils by saturating the carbon bonds chemically, and this procedure robs the oil of its metabolic advantages. Another variable of fatty acid structure is that the double bonds may have one of two forms - cis and trans. Only the cis form functions normally in us and is the natural form. The processing of vegetable oils to produce margarine and other cooking fats increases the trans forms of the same fatty acids, an undesirable result. The altered fatty acids produced by margarine hydrogenation are potentially harmful, and probably should be avoided.

One of the least desirable foods in a store is cheap margarine. Most margarines contain milk proteins and are not suitable on the Core Diet.

The disadvantage of unsaturated carbon bonds is that they are easily oxidized, and oxidized FA's tend to be toxic. If vegetable oils are cooked at high temperature in the frying pan, or deep fryer, oxidation occurs rapidly. This is the argument against fried foods. Slow fat oxidation underlies rancidity of fat. Most oils are preserved with anti-oxidants to prevent rancidity, and this appears to be a good idea. Fresh vegetable oils (PUFA) are desirable, and if no preservatives are added, the oils should not be stored for long periods of time. Light exposure increases fat oxidation, and can be reduced by brown bottles or dark-room storage.

The only fat components that are truly essential are the fatty acids, linoleic and alpha-linoleic acids. Arachidonic acid is sometimes considered essential, but may be produced inside cells by the conversion of linoleic acid. Dietary fat is complex, and confusing. Animal fats have been associated with our major diseases, atherosclerosis, which leads us to heart attacks and strokes, to cancers of the colon and breast, and to obesity.

Fat is energy dense, supplying 9 kcal/gram. Dietary fat surplus is stored as body fat, and high fat intakes are associated with obesity, except in eskimoes who continue to follow traditional patterns of sustained hard work in extreme cold weather.

Current recommendations for fat intake are shrinking progressively from 35% of total calories to 20%. Typical American diets contain as much as 42% fat, an extravagant surplus. Our needs are supplied by 15-25 grams of fat per day, 1-2% of total calories for adults and 3% for infants. Fat intakes, close to miminal need, may be desirable, especially for those at risk of fat-related disease. Our children should be introduced to a Core Diet level of fat intake-about 20% of daily calories with 60-70% fat as poylunsaturated vegetable oil. Safflower or sunflower oil is chosen because of a high content of linoleic acid.

7.5.2 Therapeutic Fatty Acids

Many articles are now been written to recommend fish oils as therapeutic agents. There may be some benefits to children to have supplemental EPA, a fatty acid derived from fish oils. EPA may help prevent heart disease. There is epidemiological evidence that fish eaters suffer less cardiovascular disease. Eicosapentenoic acid (EPA) is given the major credit for this protective effect. EPA influences many aspects of our biochemistry - especially inflammatory mediator synthesis and fat metabolism. This is an omega-3 FA , most found in fish, especially salmon, and herring.

EPA looks useful in several directions, beyond the prevention of heart attacks and strokes. Pain-relieving, anti-inflammatory action has been demonstrated in arthritis, and migraine headaches. A recent study has shown that EPA is incorporated into immune cell membranes where it alters the immune-reacting behaviour of the cells. EPA enriched cells release less leukotriene D4 which acts to recruit more cells to a site of inflammation. Less Leukotriene B4 means less inflammation. EPA at a dose of 10 1.0 gm capsules/day improved adult patients with atopic dermatitis or eczema. Eczematous skin has elevated levels of LB4. The indications for use in children are not well known. EPA at a dose of 180-540 mg may be considered in children with eczema and those with a strong family history of elevated cholesterol, and heart disease. Olive oil may prove to equally or more effective as a source of beneficial fatty acids.

Another FA, recently popular, is gamma-linoleic acid (GLA), an omega-6 FA, derived from the oil of the evening primrose, boragte, and other plants. GLA is a first cousin of Linoleic Acid, and is usually synthesised in cells from LA. Three grams per day of primrose oil, containing both linoleic acid and GLA can reduce LDL cholesterol significantly, and may lower blood pressure. GLA also helps atopic children with exczema, and may be a good adjuct to the hypoallergenic diets, which cure these children of their disease. Beneficial effects of GLA on other brain dysfunctions have been noted, and suggest a promising area of clinical application of PUFA reprogramming. GLA may also be added to the hypoallergenic diets used to treat both children and adults with affective disorders, especially moody, hyperactive children. This is a frontier in nutritional programming with too little in the way of specific, proven applications.[23]

7.5.3 Lecithin & Acetylcholine

Lecithin has become popular for two reasons. Lecithin is an emulsifying agent, and is supposed to improve blood fat transport, reduce cholesterol, and prevent heart attack. This proposed effect has not been substantiated. EPA is better candidate for that role. The second role of lecithin, the supply of phosphatidyl choline, is more interesting and relevant. We manufacture acetylcholine, the transmitter which allows us to think, remember, and move, from choline. While we produce choline internally by biosynthesis, increased dietary choline can increase acetylcholine synthesis. It is possible that active, growing children need extra dietary choline to aid learning and memory. Again little specific information is availbale. Many parents supplement lecithin and feel positive about its effects. The principle foods contributing lecithin in our diets are eggs (yolk), liver, soybeans, wheat germ, peanuts, meat, oatmeal, wheat - all limited or excluded on the Core Diet. Rice is the major choline-containing CD food. Bottled lecithin, available for food processing, and supplemention, is usually made from soyabeans. Dietary and supplemental lecithin is a complex mixture containing varying amounts of Phosphatidyl Choline (PC). Commercial soya lecithin probably contains only 20-30% PC, and is used as an emulsifying agent in a variety of food products. The problem with lecithin supplementation is that a lot is required to increase the amount of choline available to the brain. Most granular lecithin is manufactured for soya beans. Digestive symptoms, especially extra gas and bloating may limit the use of lecithin. Choline itself can be supplemented, but too much produces the unpleasant fish odor syndrome.

7.6 The Metabolism of Nutrients

Nutrients, as sensible molecules in the body, travel to cells to function in a variety of ways. Large molecules are informative in biological systems. Small molecules are functional in biological systems. For animals, like ourselves, the fundamental equation of physical existence is:

Eat Plant & Animal Tissue---->Digest----> Synthesize Me

or   A2---->Digest----->A1---->Synthesize Me

We ingest parts of the world to turn it into ourselves. If we consider the destination of food molecules, the following format emerges:

Energy: Some nutrients, like glucose and fatty acids, are used as fuel. Our metabolism dismantles the molecule, extracting its energy to supply power for muscle action and energy to our brain. Our brain, in turn, controls the whole complex orchestration of body. With this food energy, the brain also brings the entire universe to consciousness, a fine trick of biological alchemy. Finally, some of the food energy is spent to produce heat, since we are obliged to maintain a steady-state body temperature.

A quick energy dynamics equation is:

Food Energy----> Metabolism: Action: Heat: Control: Consciousness

Structure: Nutrients supply the biochemical synthesis factories within each cell with raw material to construct and maintain our tissues. Small nutrient molecules are assembled into larger structural molecules which are assembled, in turn, into cell structure. Cells arrange themselves into cooperative, architecturally coherent communities, our organs. Organs form organ systems and these systems come together in the transcendent organization of a person's body, behavior, and mental state.

Nutrients-----> Synthesis: Anabolism: structures of
increasing complexity

Information & Control: Some nutrients are destined to become hormones, transmitters, and mediators; molecules which participate in intercellular communications networks, supply the information-processing brain, regulate whole body systems, and orchestrate patterns of immune-defense responses.

Nutrients-----> Messengers: Controllers: Regulators: Control
of increasing complexity

7.6.1 Water Balance

Water is essential to life. Water accounts for over 50-70% of our body weight. While we may consider water to be a nutrient, it really deserves special status. Life essentially consists of molecular transactions occuring in water. The molecular stream flows through us in water-based chemical complex of salts, sugars, and emulsified fats. Inadequate water ingestion or increased water loss leads to dehydration, a life-threatening deficiency. Diuresis is the increased kidney excretion of salty water and waste products. As water input increases, urine flow increases. A normal kidney controls water balance remarkably well, but is fooled by drugs and diuretic beverages.

The poetry of molecular streaming translates into a science of body-input dynamics (BID). The A1 molecules have different flow rates, different control systems, and different ranges of optimal functioning concentration. From a practical point of view, we must know something about nutrient flow rates. We start with water and require a daily input of 1.8 to 2.5 liters for adults, 0.4 to 1.0 liters for infants. Increased water loss from sweating, vomiting, and diarrhea, must be rapidly replaced by water intake or the major body dysfunction, dehydration, soon threatens existence. An infant with vomiting and diarrhea is in the most trouble with water loss, since the intake requirement is high, their ability to conserve water by reducing urine production is limited, and they have no direct control of their liquid intake. Replacement of the infant's lost body fluids must include salts with water so that the concentration of electrolyte in blood and cellular fluid remains constant.

7.6.2 Nutrient Intake Goals

The destination of all nutrients is the intracellular assembly lines which require all raw materials to be present simultaneously. Naive statements, like "Vitamin A is good for your vision," should be reserved for preschool nutritional instruction. This is like recommending "rubber" to Ford Motor Company as "good for their production line". It is much more satisfying to think of the trillions of biosynthetic events per hour which keep you going and to develop a good feeling for the molecular flow supplying raw material and catalytic substances to this busy living machinery.

The NP idea is to establish a range of nutrient intakes as a guideline for adjusting food selection and designing supplement programs. The baseline values are the Recommended Daily Allowances (RDA). The RDA is an evolving committee-style guesstimate of adequate nutrient intake. The data supporting the committee decisions has been the best available, but is not yet adequate for definitive nutrient recommendations. [24] The 1980 edition of recommended dietary allowances [25] prefaced the recommendations:

> "RDA are recommendations for the average daily amounts of nutrients that population groups should consume over a period of time. RDA should not be confused with requirements for specific individuals. Differences in the nutrient requirements of individuals are ordinarily unknown...the RDA values are recommendations established for healthy populations. Special needs for nutrients arising from such problems as premature birth, inherited metabolic disorders, infections, chronic disease, and the use of medications require special dietary and therapeutic measures. These conditions are not covered by RDA."

Well-formulated diets with total calories in excess of 3000 Kcal per day tend to supply all vitamins and minerals at RDA levels and higher. Children's diets with smaller quantities of food and calories are more prone to deficiencies. As the total caloric intake drops, nutrient deficiencies begin to appear, although the overall effect of the food choices may be quite positive. One of the dogmas of standard dietetics is that all nutrients should be obtained from food. The recommendation to increase food intake sufficient to achieve RDA levels of nutrients may be counterproductive. The prescription of a reasonable nutrient supplement permits food selection, free of this nutrient-deficiency concern. The early phases of a core diet program may be deficient in a few micronutrients as indicated earlier in this chapter. Proper supplementation is a safe, cost-effective, intelligent way to assure optimal nutrient intake without compromising safe food choices.

Most dieticians need very simple rules and follow the RDA guidebook. Clients are advised to eat food from the traditional four food groups to achieve nutrient concentrations up to the RDA levels. The RDA nutrient values are based on a low-end estimate, the amount of the nutrient which prevents deficiency disease. RDA has some allowance for error and individual variation, but not enough.

If, for example, you were convinced that the data at hand suggested that 20 mg of Vitamin C/day would prevent scurvy, you would recommend that everyone ingest at least 40 mg/day to be on the safe side. Later, you may learn that Vitamin C (VM.C) is destroyed by storage and cooking, and that food estimates of Vitamin C content may mislead your trusting clients. You raise the RDA to account for food variation to 60 mg/day. Then you realize that various factors, such as smoking and drugs, interfere with the metabolism of vitamin C and you adjust upwards to 100-200 mg/day for individuals at risk. Then Linus Pauling suggests important benefits from much higher doses, 1000-5000 mg/day. You are skeptical, but eventually test the idea with disappointing but not entirely negative results. Norman Cousins publicly cures himself with high doses of Vitamin C intravenously and funny videos and becomes a professor at UCLA. Others advocate new reasons for higher doses, like the antioxidant effect of VM.C or the stomach cancer protective effect. Still others boldly treat cancer or AIDS patients with huge intravenous doses of VM.C, up to 100,000 mg/day! Now we are very far away from the RDA and only are reassured by one realization: even huge doses of VM.C are well tolerated.

The range of actual "recommended" use of Vitamin C is 60-100,000 mg/day! Whose advice are you going to follow?

One of the most persuasive arguments for the use of extra VM.C over a lifetime is its ability to scavenge free oxygen radicals. Cellular combustion can be compared to a stove, which needs adequate protection to do its job without burning the house down. As we burn fuel in our cells, some oxygen atoms are given an extra electron and become the radical, $O2-$. Oxygen will also combine with hydrogen in the free hydroxyl radical $-OH$ or in the highly reactive hydrogen peroxide molecule, $H2O2$. If $O2-$ floats free of the energy engines, it may interact vigorously with other molecules. Cell membranes are vulnerable to $O2-$ injury; damaged membranes disturb the function of the entire cell. Extra $O2-$ reacting with DNA can make the code sticky and can cause mistakes in code reading or replication, resulting in cell-mutation. The cumulative damage of trillions of random $O2-$ encounters with critical molecules over many years contributes to accelerated aging and cellular dysfunction, like cancer. Cells contain oxygen detoxification enzymes: peroxidases, superoxide dismutase, and catalases. Several molecules combine harmlessly with $O2-$ and are referred to as "antioxidants". VM.C is the cheapest, safest, and best antioxidant in town. If you can raise the amount of VM.C in cells, you may soak up enough $O2-$'s to make a long-term difference. The effect of VM.C is enhanced if you present two other nutrient antioxidants alongside, VM.E and selenium. You cannot take superoxide dismutase by mouth and expect benefit, since it will not arrive at the intracellular locations where it it needed. Intravenous injection of the enzyme may, however, be an effective treatment of inflammatory disorders.

I was alarmed to read a newpaper story showing the singer, Michael Jackson, sleeping in a hyperbaric chamber. The newspaper article claimed that Michael was seeking increased longevity from the supersaturated oxygen atmosphere the hyperbaric chamber provides. The oxygen-free radical theory would predict the opposite result - accelerated tissue damage from the extra oxygen. This problem is already appreciated in premature infants, kept in oxygenated incubators. The high concentrations of oxygen may damage the infants' lungs. Vitamin E, another good antioxidant, protects these infants from this damage. All essential substances are needed in rather precise concentrations. Too much may be as damaging as too little.

7.6.3 Active Transport of Nutrients

The RDA of several nutrients may not be sufficient if the mechanism of absorption is impaired. Many nutrients are selectively and carefully carried across the bowel wall by enzyme systems. This active transport is the input regulator to body space. Some A1's - vitamin B12 for example - have rather complicated journeys to make; B12 requires a transport molecule, called intrinsic factor, before It can be actively transported across the small bowel wall. If you lack Intrinsic factor, oven large amounts of B12 in your diet will not help you avoid pernicious anemia, the overt B12 deficiency disease. Without intrinsic factor, B12 shots are needed to get the vitamin inside. Sodium, potassium, iron, and calcium are all actively transported minerals. Amino acids and fatty acids are also actively transported.

An important principle of NP is that each person has an individual best fit. Many of the decisions made about nutrient quantity make sense only if you have stabilized and balanced your diet, assessed it by a computed nutritional analysis, and then supplemented selected nutrients to achieve a desirable range of values. Normal functioning and normal laboratory-measured body parameters confirm that nutrient absorption matches the estimate of nutrient intake.

7.6.4 Biochemical Individuality

The problem with RDA is that there are so many variables in the nutrient-intake equation that they cannot be predicted without more specific information about individuals. One of the most important considerations is that we are all different biochemically. Nutritional advice, generated by committees for large populations of people, is not the advice that individuals, exercising personal perogatives, want for the realization of personal health goals.

Dr. Donald Davis states:[26]

> "The concept that individual differences in nutrient requirements may have unsuspected implications for the broad fields of health and medicine was first proposed in 1950 by Roger Williams...A large body of experimental data...leads to the unavoidable conclusion that individual variations of 2-,5-,or 10-fold or more, commonly exist in normal human populations...Also recognized are rare abnormal Individuals who require some 100 to 1000 times greater than average amounts of a particular nutrient due to serious inborn errors of metabolism."

There is no specific technology which allows us to define individual nutrient needs. Even the measurement of vitamin levels in the blood is an expensive lab procedure, not routinely undertaken. The only serum nutrient levels I measure regularly are sodium, potassium, calcium, magnesium, iron, vitamin B12, and folic acid. Other mineral levels - copper, manganese, and zinc - are measured in unusual situations. Even knowing blood nutrient levels, we still cannot assess the concentration within cells or the metabolic effectiveness of a nutrient. Hair analysis of mineral concentrations is of little value since it raises more questions than it answers. Many indirect and complicated biochemical analyses can be performed, but are meaningful only to exceedingly clever physicians, who correlate lab data with clinical findings.

Lacking specific, affordable, readily-available metabolic assessment technologies, the Core Diet program relies on a well-tested, thoughtful approach to diet design. The parent's role is to observe their child carefully while encouraging new food introductions. Most children need a great deal of support in changing their food habits. Once an adequate intake of vegetable foods, rice, poultry and fish is established, adequate if not superior nutrition is all but established. NP advocates a thoughtful approach to individual nutrient-intake evaluation along with trials of nutrient supplementation within the optimal ranges. When children feel, function, and grow well, their nutrition is normal.

The nutrient intake goal is to achieve nutrient levels within an optimal range. While, in theory, all nutrients are best delivered in food, in practice, it is seldom possible to balance all nutrient levels within the optimal range by manipulating food choices alone. NP has no objection to taking nutrients in their pure and elemental form. Indeed, from the NP point of view, accurate body programming is most readily achieved by dealing only in crystalline-pure nutrients, not food. My prediction is that elemental nutrient formulas (ENF), custom-formulated, will be the optimal nutrition of the future. The optimal range for each nutrient is a best-guesstimate and should not be followed blindly. The ranges allow enough room to accommodate the biochemical variability of individuals. Many of the upper values permit "therapeutic" levels of the nutrients without risking toxicity.

Chapter 8

GASTROINTESTINAL TRACT: GIT

The first gastrointestinal tract (GIT) was invented by early sea animals which were little more than floating GITs, processing sea water to obtain nourishment. As animals grew larger and more complex, the GIT elongated, disappeared inside the abdomen, and developed a system of supporting organs - the liver and pancreas, for example, which supply digestive juices. Food processing or "digestion" requires mechanical mixing of food and water, chemical breakdown of large molecules into small nutrient molecules and absorption of the right stuff into the blood.

Each person's food supply must be matched to the capacity of their GIT to process food. Dysfunction and disease arises when there is a mismatch. The infant GIT cannot handle solid foods and mother's milk is only proper input to GIT for several months. As the GIT matures increase surface area, better antibody protection, increased digestive enzymes all permit solid foods to be processed succesfully. Food introduction to infants should be a slow careful testing of GIT capacity to handle foods without problems. As children grow more nutrients must be absorbed and optimal GIT function is required to achieve optimal development. Wrong food choices and/or wrong GIT processing spoil optimal development.

8.0.1 GIT Behavior

The function of the GIT is to process food. The GIT is not a passive processor of food, but, rather, it actively manages and responds to food with a peculiar kind of behavior. The GIT is muscular and contracts rhythmically to conduct food through its length (peristalsis). If the contractions are too vigorous, crampy pain is experienced. If the contractions are too frequent and vigorous, diarrhea results. Constipation occurs when contractions are sluggish and slow, or if sustained (spastic) contractions act to obstruct the GIT. When all is well, we ignore the presence of the GIT and awareness is limited to full or empty sensations. When there is trouble in the GIT, our attention is directed to the abdomen by a variety of discomforts, pain, noise, distension, and abnormal bowel movements.

8.0.2 GIT as an Immune Sensing Surface

The GIT's surface is sensitive, knowledgeable, and reactive. The sensing, deciding, acting function of the GIT is achieved by its immune-defense department which extends along the surface. The velvety surface of the GIT is described as mucosa.

A continuous sensing apparatus in the mucosa is nicknamed MALT, short for its formal title - Mucosa Associated Lymphatic Tissue. It is MALT that supervises immune response, and food allergy. MALT at the front of the GIT itches, burns, and swells, in the same way and to the same foods that MALT at the end of the GIT does.

The GIT knows when the wrong stuff has entered its space, and reacts defensively to get rid of it. Vomiting and diarrhea interrupt normal living in a distressing display of the GIT's reactivity. Often the food input to the GIT is neglected as a source of dysfunction or disease - an oversight that is a difficult to understand. If your Doctor attempts to diagnose or treat digestive and/or food allergy problems without enquiring about and changing your child's food intake, find a new Doctor.

8.1 The Function & Features of GIT

The task of the GIT is to take apart complex food molecules and to absorb simpler, safer molecules into the blood stream, both directly and indirectly, via the blood and lymphatic drainage of the GIT. All food molecules are absorbed by the GIT, mostly from the small intestine (duodenum, jejunum, ileum). After food molecules are absorbed, they are carried in the venous blood (portal veins) from the GIT to the liver. The liver's main task is to take in a large percentage of the newly absorbed food molecules for further chemical processing, storage, and slow release. The liver is a complex chemical factory, whose function is to control the food supply for the rest of the body. Food molecules leaving the liver are distributed throughout the body in the bloodstream.

8.1.1 Digestive Secretions

Digestion of food is accomplished by secretions from the bowel surface and glands accessory to the bowel. The liver and pancreas are the major secretory organs which contribute digestive factors to the bowel. The first digestive secretions are produced by the salivary glands which secrete into our mouth. Saliva is a lubricant watery fluid, containing amylase, an enzyme which reduces starch into its component sugars. If you chew starchy food for any length of time, you may experience increasing sweetness as amylase liberates individual sugar molecules from the starch polymer. Saliva is a prototype of all the digestive juices secreted by the GIT. Its secretion is controlled by nerves of the autonomic nervous system, and varies with smells, sight, sounds, and emotions. Activity in the sympathetic and parasympathetic nerves increases salivary secretion; drugs which block this activity will produce a dry mouth (eg. drugs used to treat colic or cramps). Saliva contains antibodies, especially IgA, as the first line of immune defense against ingested noxious substances.

8.1.2 Stomach Action

Digestion continues in the stomach, which mixes the food by strong muscular action with strong hydrochloric acid (HCl) produced by the parietal cells lining the stomach surface. More enzymes are secreted by the stomach:

1. Renin, which coagulates milk.

2. Pepsinogen, which is activated by acid to become pepsin which, in turn, breaks down large protein molecules into smaller chains called polypeptides.

3. Lipase, which breaks down fat molecules.

The lining of the stomach is protected from its own acid by surface factors including mucus and prostaglandins. If the surface defence breaks down, hydrochloric acid may erode the surface of the stomach or the first part of the small bowel (duodenum), producing a "peptic" ulcer.

8.1.3 The Small Intestine

Partly-digested, well-mixed food is squeezed out of the stomach through an outlet valve, the pylorus, into the small intestine. The small intestine is a coiled muscular GIT which does most of the chemical work of digesting and absorbing food. The liver produces bile as its contribution to digestion. Bile flows into the duodenum via a tubular system with a storage sac, the gall bladder, connected by a T-junction. Beyond the duodenum is the jejunum where nutrients are derived from food and absorbed. Absorption is completed in the third section of intestine, the ileum. The ileum delivers a watery slurry of leftover food waste to the colon or large intestine.

8.1.4 Gall Bladder

The gall bladder is simply a muscular sac which stores bile secreted by the liver, and releases it in gushes when eating stimulates gall bladder contraction. The action of the gall bladder is regulated by gut hormones, particularly cholecystokinin, released by the stimulation of the small intestine by food molecules. Fat is a particularly strong stimulus for the contraction of the gall bladder. A low fat diet is recommended for anyone with stones in the gall bladder, to reduce the likelihood of strong contractions which might push stones into the bile duct causing the very severe pain of biliary colic.

8.1.5 Bile

The liver secretion, bile, is the yellow bitter fluid which you may have occasionally seen and tasted when you have vomited. It also provides the yellow pigment, bilirubin, which produces jaundice in a variety of abnormal circumstances. Bile contains a complex mixture of chemicals which participate in the digestion of food. The role of bile salts is to emulsify or break-up fat into small droplets and suspend these droplets in the water. Once fat is suspended as small droplets in the bowel soup, fat-cleaving enzymes, the pancreatic lipases, can dissociate the larger fat molecules into their component molecules, fatty acids and glycerol.

The emulsion of fat droplets is absorbed by the microvilli of the small intestine, where intestinal cells perform complicated processing on the fat molecules before releasing their products into the intestinal lymph or directly into the portal venous circulation. The details of fat molecule transformation are exceeding complex. Because fat absorption and blood fat transport require such highly sophisticated cellular chemistry, there is enormous opportunity for things to go wrong. Fat overload in our diets is a principle risk factor for blood vessel disease (atherosclerosis), and is a major contributor to obesity in those who overeat. The Core Diet is a very low fat program which could be prescribed to reduce the risk of obesity, coronary artery disease, and strokes.

8.1.6 Pancreas

The pancreas contributes many enzymes to the small intestine to process food. Deficiency of pancreatic enzymes prevents proper digestion and diarrhea associated with fat loss in the liquid stool (steatorrhea) ensues. People with Cystic Fibrosis have pancreatic enzyme deficiency and suffer diarrhea with malabsorption of essentialnutrients. Pancreatic enzymes are secreted as inactive molecules (zymogens), which must be converted in the alkaline environment of the small intestine to active substances. The active enzymes break down large protein molecules into smaller components - short chains of amino acids, called peptides, or amino acids themselves.

The pancreatic enzymes are trypsin, chymotrypsin, elastase, and carboxypeptidases. The wall of the small intestine produces the rest of the enzymes necessary to digest food. The intestinal proteinase, enterokinase, is essential for the activation of the pancreatic proenzymes. Each enzyme prefers to work on specific areas of proteins or peptides. Maximal absorption of tracer-labelled protein in a test meal has been found as early as 45 minutes after ingestion. This rapid absorption means that some protein is absorbed before complete digestion can be achieved. Peptide absorption may have profound physiogical and pathological significance - the most serious forms of food allergy are triggered by wrong entry of proteins and/or peptides.

Digestion and absorption of nutrients is completed in the small intestine, and a semiliquid waste material is then delivered to the large intestine, or colon, where water is absorbed and, in normal circumstances, a solid waste product is formed and stored for later evacuation.

8.1.7 The Colon

The colon is a complex and somewhat mysterious organ. The colon can be compared to a septic tank, distinguished by its unpleasant contents - fermenting, putrifying food-wastes. Trillions of microorganisms live in the colon, many of which are exceedingly dangerous if let loose in the body.

The "septic" compartment is useful for the further degradation of undigested food, and the liberation of some nutrients. We are no longer dependent on colon microorganisms for nutrients like vitamin K and biotin, and could theoretically give up the septic function of the colon. It proves almost impossible, however, to reduce microorganism growth in the colon. All the hopeful people who seek colon cleanliness with enemas, laxatives, purges, and herbs are engaged in a futile, and sometimes counterproductive, exercise. Enteros, the space inside the GIT, remains "outside" the body. If the contents of the colon are spilled into the abdomen by a perforated bowel, a life-threatening infection, peritonitis, ensues.

The colon's dense population of microorganisms is important to us in health and disease. The bacteria feed on undigested carbohydrate. 99% of them survive best in the absence of oxygen (anaerobic bacteria). It is estimated that 10-15% of starch from cereal grains and potatoes and up to 50% of milk sugar enter the colon undigested, where they are fermented by colon bacteria. Many vegetables contain undigestible carbohydrate which is welcomed by the colon flora. The gas associated with beans is produced by the fermentation of these carbohydrates. Colon fermentation produces hydrogen gas, which may distend the bowel and produce pain. Methane and carbon dioxide are other odorless gases produced by fermentation. The foul smells of colon gas are mostly volatile substances produced by the putrifaction of undigested protein, and indicate a maldigestive state. Many chemical substances are produced by colon bacteria and may be absorbed into the body. Some products are desirable, like vitamin K and biotin. Other products are nutrients, like fatty acids, which supply a small percentage of the calories extracted from food. Yet other substances produced in the colon may be undesirable; these include alcohols, lactic acid, and formate. The unpleasant smelling colonic gases are also absorbed and excreted by the lungs, giving the exhaled breath an unpleasant smell (halitosis). No amount of mouthwash, gum, or widely advertised candies will alter malodorous breath, but diet revision can correct the problem.

The role of the colon as a metabolic organ is not well understood. One important metabolic role is the regulation of the body ammonia burden. Ammonia (NH_3) is derived from dietary protein, the principle source of nitrogen in the body. Nitrogen freed from protein breakdown is toxic and must be excreted. Ammonia poisoning may occur in a variety of circumstances, especially liver disease. Subtle degrees of ammonia intoxication may be a common cause of brain dysfunction.

A generous intake of dietary fiber, as undigestible carbohydrate, aids colon bacteria in incorporating ammonia in their own structure and metabolism, and results in a lower body ammonia burden. Diets, deficient in fibre and high in protein produce the opposite effect - increased body burden of ammonia. Patients suffering liver disease with elevated blood ammonia are improved by the oral intake of lactulose, an undigestible carbohydrate which increases bacterial protein synthesis. One can use the sniff-test to assess the colon's protein-carbohydrate balance: smelly gas reveals increased protein putrefaction, and may be associated with increased body ammonia, whereas non-odorous gas indicates healthier carbohydrate fermentation.

The secret of good colon function is a healthy balanced population of microorganisms. When colon ecology is disturbed, there is a heavy penalty to pay. Evidence is accumulating that immune responses to colon bacteria antigens may play a role in the production of serious disease like Rheumatoid Arthritis. Disturbed colon ecology is associated with diarrhea, and may cause ulcerative colitis. Antibiotics may cause major disturbances in colon ecology and occasionally cause a life-threatening overgrowth of toxic bacteria ("Necrotising enterocolitis").

8.1.8 Oral Effects of Food Reactions

Food allergy is first declared in the mouth. Our mouths are full of immune monitoring information. If we are willing to tune into the sensations originating from oral sensors, sensitive, subtle signs of food reactions may be picked up in the mouth, before more major trouble begins further along the GIT, or systemically in body space. (If only patients and physicians alike would pay attention!). Swelling reactions of the lips, tongue, and throat express the most dramatic and serious type of allergic responses of MALT. As offending, allergenic molecules pass through the mouth, surface antibodies, attached to mast cells, react with the food antigens. The mast cell reaction produces swelling and inflammation of the lips, mouth surfaces, and throat. The reaction may be minute, limited to swelling of a small area on the tongue, or may cause a life-threatening swelling of the whole tongue and throat. Small ulcers (aphthous ulcers) are common consequences of an allergic reaction. Painful sensations are common as nerve endings of the tongue, mouth, and throat are stimulated by inflammatory mediators. Abnormal taste sensations are commonly reported, including a generalized blunting of taste. The tongue feels coated, or tastes abnormally, often detecting a metallic taste, which may persist long after the offending substances are ingested.

Continuous allergic inflammation in the mouth and nose may obliterate pleasant eating sensations and is associated with disordered food selection. The complete sensation of taste is dependent on proper smell, obliterated by a stuffy, swollen nose. People in this predicament often opt for heavy doses of the primary tastes, salt and sugar. The taste-impaired lose interest in more healthy foods with subtle flavors (especially vegetables), since they cannot perceive the tastes. This blunting of flavor sensation is one of the routes to faulty food selection, picky and compulsive eating.

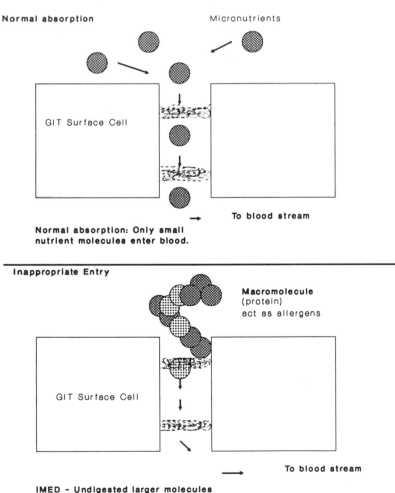

Normal absorption   Micronutrients

GIT Surface Cell

To blood stream

Normal absorption: Only small
nutrient molecules enter blood.

Inappropriate Entry

Macromolecule
(protein)
act as allergens

GIT Surface Cell

To blood stream

IMED - Undigested larger molecules
enter blood to cause food allergy.

Chapter 9
FOOD ADDITIVES AND CONTAMINANTS

9.1 Food Additives

Food additives are chemicals used at home or by the food industry to improve the taste, color, texture, and longevity of food. Food preservation with salt, smoke, spices, and sugars is the origin of food additive technology. Commercial food additives are regulated in the U.S.A. by the Federal Food, Drug, and Cosmetic Act. Food additives tend to receive the most detailed scientific attention because of regulatory scrutiny. We know far less about the chemicals intrinsic to food than we know about additives. An excellent review of food additives and their regulation can be found in "Foodborne Disease & Food Safety" by Angela Gilchrist.[27] A handy reference is the "Food Additives Book".[28] A handy technical reference is "Food Additives" by Thomas Furia.[29] A brief discussion of the more popularly problematic additives will serve to illustrate problems related to additives.

9.1.1 Sulphites

Sulphites are used as bleaching, antioxidant, and preserving additives in food. Increasingly, sulphites have been implicated as allergens. A typical sulphite reaction involves flushing, dizziness, shortness of breath or wheezing. Asthmatic attacks can be provoked by sulphites and a few deaths have been attributed to them. Sulphite sprays have been widely used on fresh produce in stores and restaurants to prevent browning with air exposure. French-fried potatoes are also treated this way. As preservatives, sulphites were found in processed food, alcoholic beverages (wines and beer), and drugs. Even aerosols used to treat asthmatics contained sulphites as preservatives! The increased notoriety of sulphites in 1985 has led new regulations limiting their use. The FDA has banned the use of six sulphite preservatives in fresh fruit and vegetables. The ban still permits manufacturers of processed foods, dried fruits, wines and beer to use sulphites, although, if these manufacturers are prudent, they will voluntarily restrain or curtail sulphite use.

9.1.2 Nitrites

Nitrites, usually sodium salts, have been used widely as preservatives, especially in bacon and other processed meats. Saltpeter is the best known nitrite with its undeserved reputation as the sex-drive inhibitor. Nitrites also occur naturally in foods. The chief concern is the ability of nitrites to combine with amino acids in the bowel to form nitrosamines, potentially carcinogenic molecules. Vitamin C inhibits nitrosamine formation and is thought to protect against GIT cancer. Vitamin C is an antioxidant preservative, and can replace less desirable preservatives in some foods. Tobacco smoke is the major source of human exposure to nitrosamines.[30]

9.1.3 Salicylates

The world's most used drug is acetylsalicylic acid (ASA), or aspirin, the grandmother of salicylates. Other salicylates are common in vegetables and fruit; the first medicinal salicylates came from plant sources like willow bark. Methylsalicylate has been rubbed on many cold-stricken chests and inhaled freely by coughing children, with all the conviction of recovery that mothers' best medicine can convey. In its prime, ASA was found in hundreds of over-the-counter medications and was associated with pain relief more than any other drug in history. ASA is an effective drug, with diverse benefits, but it routinely causes GIT irritation and bleeding. It is a good allergen, and causes many rashes and hives. Salicylates ocassionally trigger asthma and have been implicated in deaths from respiratory failure. The implication of ASA in Reye's Syndrome, a rare, but sometimes fatal, allergic-type reaction following viral illnesses, has led to widespread substitution of acetaminophen as a pain-reliever, with fever-reducing characteristics. Dr. Feingold postulated that salicylates and food dyes produced hyperactivity in children, and popularized low salicylate diets. These chemicals have not proven to be the most important causes of childrens' behavioral disorders, although they remain a potential problem and must be considered whenever food problems present. Feingold recommended avoiding foods that contained natural salicylates or chemically similar substances. His lists excluded such foods as peaches and cucumber, for example, which are low in our list of symptom-producing foods.

9.1.4 Food Dyes and Preservatives

Food colors and preservatives have been suspected of producing allergic reactions, and behavioral disturbance. Their exclusion was part of Dr. Feingold's program for treating hyperactive children. Food colors are used liberally in all commercial food manufacture and have been popular in home use. The yellow dye, tartrazine, is definitely associated with hives (urticaria), as is the preservative, benzoate. In the study of hyperactive children by Egger et al, tartrazine and benzoate were the commonest substances to provoke abnormal behavior in children, although they were never the only cause of behavioral problems.

Tartrazine is a yellow food color, common in a wide variety of manufactured food products. Tartrazine produces symptoms typically within 90 minutes of eating producing a variety of symptoms, including asthma, hives, generalized swelling, headache, and behavior change, usually hyperactivity. Colors derived from natural plant and animal sources are usually exempt from FDA control and are generally recognized as safe (GRAS). Beet pigment, beta-carotene, grape skin extract, paprika, saffron, turmeric, and vegetable juice are example of GRAS colors. While these substances are not known to be toxic, nor carcinogenic, there is no assurance that they are not allergenic, or otherwise troublesome to some people. Certified colors are approved by the Food Drug and Cosmetic act and bear the certification name FD&C Red No. 2 and so on. Tartrazine is FD&C Yellow No. 15. Of the nine colors currently certified, seven may be used in amounts consistent with good manufacturing practice.

9.1.5 Monosodium Glutamate

Monosodium Glutamate, well-known as MSG, is perhaps the most villified of additives. MSG is blamed for almost everything that goes wrong in a Chinese restaurant, and many people scan food product labels, rejecting any bold enough to display MSG. It is likely that MSG is a victim of the single ingredient fallacy, discussed in earlier chapters. Ironically, glutamate is a perfectly respectable, normal amino acid, continuously present in all our cells, and always available in the blood. One possibility for MSG to act in a negative fashion would occur with the sudden absorption of a large amount. A rapid rise in blood glutamate may activate receptors which ring alarms, causing the headache and shooting pains that are associated with MSG. A variety of other symptoms are commonly reported, including flushing, numbness and tingling, cheat pains, fast heart action, abdominal pains and behavior changes, including irritablity, hyperactivity, and angry outbursts. In pure form, we would not expect MSG to trigger allergic effects. MSG products may contain allergenic contaminants from the vegetable source including corn, beets, and wheat. Often MSG is mixed with an enzyme in commercial food enhancers like "Accent". The most common enzyme is Papain, derived from Papaya. Papain is a protein allergen. It is possible that MSG is often blamed for the allergenicity of papain. Papain may be injected into ruptured intervertebral discs as an alternative to back surgery. The injection is potentially dangerous if the patient has been previously sensitized to papain by ingestion of it in food. This risk illustrates the immune principle that ingestion of an allergen may sensitize the whole body to its effects. We are immunized against the food we eat. Skin testing does not predict all papain reactions, but should precede any attempt to inject it into the body.

9.1.6 Aspartame

The popular artifical sweetener, aspartame, contains two normal amino acids - phenylalanine and aspartic acid. The sweetness of this combination was a suprise discovery. The ingestion of this substance should pose little or no problem to many children, except children with phenylalanine intolerance.

9.2 Contaminants and Carcinogens

Briefly, let us consider one of the unhappy facts of the 20th century. Our food supply is contaminated by a variety of agricultural chemicals, water and air pollutants. We are told that we must live with a degree of chemical contamination, since our industrialized, agricultural industry depends on chemical technology to feed us. Predatory insects threaten the farmer's economic existence, and it is easy to understand why the insects are sprayed until dead. The replacement of long-lived with shorter-lived chemicals is in our favor, but hardly reassures us when we become ill with ill-defined-illness. Organic gardening appeals on all levels of value except practicality. The expectation of attractive, relatively uniform-looking produce demands an industrialized agriculture with an efficient protection and preservation technology. Less hazardous insect-control methods have been proposed. The biological control of insects is an improving technology, and may eventually rescue us from self-inflicted poisoning.

The major contaminants in our food supply are:

* Pesticides, herbicides, and fungicides
* Antibiotics and hormones in animal tissues
* Environmental contaminants, including toxic heavy
* Metals – lead and mercury
* Radioactive isotopes
* Organic acids,
* Hydrocarbon residues (from fuel combustion)
* Processing, refining contaminants, detergents,
* Bleaching agents, solvent residues, waxes, dyes
* Biological contaminants – endotoxins
* Insect and parasite eggs, rodent feces
* Bacteria, fungi, and viruses
* Contaminants from shipping and storage containers

9.2.1 Pesticides

My environmental awareness was awaked by Rachel Carson's "Silent Spring", which I recall reading serially in the New Yorker, as an impressionable adolescent. I have been on the side of the environment ever since. At that time, the major ecological poison was DDT, a long-lasting chlorinated hydrocarbon which stayed in the food chain, poisoning birds, animals, and people for many years. DDT had its benevolent side, especially in the reduction of malaria-carrying mosquitoes in tropical countries. The persistent reliance of agricultural on poisonous chemicals has mortgaged our ecosystem with a very high interest rate. Farm workers are immediately at risk of chemical poisoning, although the danger they face is often minimized or denied by "authorities" and chemical vendors. People living downwind of sprayed fields and orchards are vulnerable. People who eat chemically contaminated plants and animals are also also vulnerable.

Individual sensitivity to chemicals varies greatly, and is interactive with other chemical stressors. The biological effects of agricultural chemicals are not so well-known that any authority can assure you all is well. Chronic exposure to low doses of chemicals is likely to lead to chronic illness. People who use insecticides at home on a regular basis also risk toxicity and should reconsider this use. I have seen several patients who became sick after their houses were fumigated for fleas, termites, cockroaches, or ants. They were reassured that there would be no problem. The reassurance consists only of the ignorance and wishful thinking of the pest control vendor, who, after all, has to make his living too.

The effect of agricultural chemical contamination of the food supply is not known. Dr. Laseter has reported[31] finding pesticides in the blood of 200 sick patients who suffer environmental sensitivity. DDT was found in 62%, hexacholobenzene in 57.5%, Heptachlor epoxide in 54%, Beta-BHC in 34%, Endosulfan in 34%, Dieldrin in 24%, and Chlordane in 20%. Other pesticides were also found. Only 1% of the patients tested were free of pesticides!

9.2.2 Dioxins

Dioxins are group of highly toxic chlorinated hydrocarbons, originating in agricultural and industrial chemicals and persisting in the environment for many years. PCB's (polychlorinated biphenyls) are the best known source of dioxins. PCB's have been used extensively since the 1930's. Swedish scientists first noted PCB's in birds in 1966. Since then, many studies have documented the existence of PCB's in animals, plants, and fresh water supplies. Recent spills of PCB's from transformers in electrical systems have been newsworthy reminders of dioxin hazards.

The herbicide-defoliant Agent Orange gained notoriety after its extensive use in Vietnam. Its most toxic component is TCDD (tetrachlorodibenzo-para-dioxin). Dr. Schecter[32] reported finding alarmingly high levels of TCDD in the breast milk of American and Canadian mothers. Evidently, dioxins are widely distributed in our food supply, and are stored in the fat of our bodies, once ingested. Elevated dioxin levels have been found in poultry, pork, beef, milk, eggs, and fish. Dr. Shecter was quoted:

> "Breast-fed infants represent a population with daily exposure to dioxins and related chemicals and I am very concerned about the potential health effects at the levels we found."

9.2.3 Alar and Apples

Alar is a chemical (daminozide) sprayed on apple orchards to keep ripening apples on the trees and to improve appearance of the apple after picking. The U.S. Environmental Protection Agency proposed a ban on Alar which was subsequently withdrawn - they had evidence of a cancer-causing effect of a breakdown product UDMH. Apple juice was especially suspect because the heat used in juice production created UDMH. Shortly after Consumer Reports published an article on Alar,[33] its manufacturer, Uniroyal, withdrew it from the market. The article states:

> "Consumers, especially parents, should not accept Alar in the apple juice and should not be required to rely on industry promises that aren't always kept...it's the governments job to protect all consumers. The EPA should ban daminozide sooner rather than later."

9.2.4 Coping with Dangers of Agricultural Chemicals

What does the presence of industrial and agricultural chemicals in our childrens' tissues mean? If you have a toxin in your body, which should not be there, what assumption are you going to make? These chemicals are good metabolic poisons, and so you are going to assume that they will in some way alter the way your body works. Right off the bat, agricultural chemical residues in the body mean increased risk of illness until proven otherwise. The people who deny the problem (until proven otherwise) are not credible.

Pesticides have a special proclivity to alter the way our brain works and, therefore, the way we think, feel, remember, and act.[34] The same chemicals tend to intefere with immune functions, so you are going to assume that immune surveillance will be compromised, which means that you may get more infectious illness, and have a higher risk of cancer. Rather than despairing, there are practical steps to be taken individually and collectively to reduce the pollution hazard.

Vegetables and fruit should be washed in hot water, and peeled before use. Efforts to control insect predators by safer biological methods should receive generous support. Better chemical monitoring of produce is desirable. Farmers should be rewarded for their efforts to reduce chemical contamination of their crops. More research is needed to survey the extent of chemical contamination of our bodies, and its consequences. The immediate adverse effects of pesticides should be better appreciated in clinical medicine, and methods of detoxifiction should be developed and employed as routine therapy.

9.2.5 Heavy Metals

Lead is the major heavy-metal contaminant to find its way into our food supply in increasing amounts. US industry consumes 1.3 million metric tons of lead annually, releasing half of it into the environment each year. Leaded fuels contribute 90% to air lead pollution, and have increased the agricultural burden of lead. Soils contaminated by airborne lead accumulate the mineral, and plants absorb it from the soil. Increasing acidity of soils from fertilizers and acid rain increase the solubility of heavy metals like lead. Animals grazing on leaded plants concentrate the mineral in their bones. People eating leaded plants, eating soups made with boiled bones, or supplementing their calcium intake with bone meal increase their lead intake. Lead poisoning from food ingestion alone is seldom apparent, but will contribute to the body burden of problems. The introduction of lead-free gasoline has had good effects, with avergage blood lead levels in US citizens dropping 37% between 1976 and 1980.[35] The decline of the Roman empire has been attributed to lead poisoning from the popularity of pewter dishware, containing lead, and lead-lined water conduits. Increased water acidity may have increased lead's toxicity to the Romans as it threatens our own populations exposed to acid rain. The shift of mineral absorption of crops exposed to acid rain is one of the many imponderables of our food supply - a variable which can shift the metabolic norms of whole populations.

Mecury poisoning has appeared tragically in people who ingested large amounts of mercury-contaminated fish. The Japanese experience with mercury poisoning was an example for the rest of the world. Mercury levels in free-swimming ocean fish do not appear to be a problem. Bottom-feeding fish near sources of industrial mercury pollution are the high-risk food sources.

9.2.6 Chlorine and Fluorides

The concern about ill effects of chlorinated water has a legitimacy which the concern about fluoride supplemention has not. Municipal water supplies are commonly disinfected with chlorine gas or hypochlorite salts, which liberate free chlorine. Chlorine is definitely a toxic gas, as anyone who uses chlorine bleach at close quarter knows. Chlorine combines with organic matter in water to form chloramines and other troublesome substances. Many people report symptoms when they ingest significant quantities of chlorinated water, and feel better when they switch to distilled or spring water. The mechanism of this adverse reaction remains obscure. Obvious toxicity symptoms also occur in people who frequent chlorinated swimming pools, whirlpool baths, and hot-tubs. Eye and respiratory irritation are easily attributed to this exposure. Less obvious is the appearance of ill-defined illness in these people, where chlorine exposure is probably acting synergistically with other stressor molecules to produce illness.

Chloride is distinct from chlorine and can be considered an essential nutrient. Sodium Chloride (NaCl) is normal table salt. Life consists of molecular transactions occuring in a salt solution - water and sodium chloride in a concentration of slighly less than 1%. Fluoride bears the same relation to Fluorine and Chloride to chlorine. The addition of sodium fluoride to drinking water to prevent dental caries has been one of the most hotly debated public health issues. The fluoride salt bears no chemical relationship to fluorine gas in the free state, which is unquestionably toxic. In the correct micro-dosage, fluoride is considered an essential nutrient. Fluoride does increase the hardness of tooth enamel, and protects against tooth decay. Fluoride supplementation is also recommended to prevent osteoporosis, and is a more legitimate bone-growth stimulator than is calcium. In excess, fluoride causes tooth mottling in children. Proper dosage is essential to obtain the benefits of fluoride without toxicity.

9.2.7 Radioactivity

The explosion of the Chernobyl nuclear reactor, April 1986, reminded the world of the omnipresent risk of radioactive contamination of our ecosystem. Nuclear weapons testing and reactor accidents contaminate the entire planet. Some long-lived radioactive isotopes are concentrated in the food chain, and remain a problem of our food and water supply for decades. Calls from worried mothers and pregnant women, seeking my advice about iodine supplements and food choices, renewed my sense of immediacy of the radiation problem, which years of complacency have obscured. The open-air testing of nuclear weapons introduced the first new load of isotopes into our ecosytem with demonstrable ill effects. Studies after the Three Mile Island accident in March 1979 demonstrated an early increase in cancer incidence in people living atop adjacent hills. The rising radioactive cloud exposed these people to primary radiation. It is postulated that the radioactivity impaired their immune defence, and cancers already existing in them then grew unchecked to produce clinically apparent disease. The appearance of cancer, newly induced by radiation, is usually delayed many years if the dose is small. The Chernobyl incident demonstrates the early inclusion of isotopes into the food chain, with increased radiation levels found almost immediately in leafy greens growing in contaminated fields, and in cows' milk. Rain becomes radioactive. Cisterns collecting rain for drinking water are immediately suspect. Soils contaminated by radioactive fallout produce crops with increased radioactivity for years to come. Animals grazing on contaminated fields will concentrate isotopes, like strontium-90, in their tissues, and will pass the isotopes on to the carnivore who eats them. Plutonium, with a half-life of 24,000 years, is the most dangerous isotope produced in nuclear reactors.

Radioactive iodine, I-131, competes with dietary supplies of normal iodine, and may be concentrated and stored in the thyroid gland. I-131 has a short half-life of 8 days, and poses only an immediate danger to those directly exposed to radioactive fallout. Concentration and storage of the isotope in the thyroid increases the risk of cell mutation, and the subsequent emergence of cancer. Immediate impairment of thyroid function may also occur. Supplements of iodine reduce the opportunity for the radioactive isotope to be taken up. Doses as high as 100 mg of potassium iodide for 7-10 days have been recommended for those directly exposed to radioactive fallout. This is a toxic dose of iodide under normal circumstances, and should not be taken unless there is real danger. The principle of nutrient supplementation to compete with uptake of radioactive isotopes is usually not considered as an indication for nutrient supplementation, and may be an important consideration for all of us.

Strontium-90 has accumulated in the food chain from weapons testing, and is concentrated in animal and fish bones. The slow accumulation of this isotope, with a half-life of 20 years, can be expected to increase the mutation rate in bone and bone marrow, increasing the incidence of bone cancer and leukemia. Calcium supplemention may compete with strontium-90 and reduce its storage. Radioactive calcium-45 is also produced by fission; with a half-life of 164 days, it is a shorter term concern, but is another condition for full calcium supplementation in populations exposed to radioactive contamination. Cesium-137, with a half-life of 33 years, is also a concern, and is distributed throughout the body, taking the place of potassium. Radioactive carbon, with a half life of 5700 years, is distributed throughout the living world, and offers no opportunity for competitive defense.

Some nutrients, especially the antioxidants, offer some protection against radioactive damage. The principle mechanism of cellular damage is ionization, the production of charged free radicals which behave abnormally in molecular transactions. The effects of ionization are most pronounced when the delicate mechanisms of DNA replication and repair are damaged. The result is cellular dysfunction, and mutation of the genetic program. A complete antioxidant formula offers meager protection and includes vitamin C 1000-5000 gm, vitamin E 400-1200 IU, selenium 200 ug, cystine 250mg - ?, and vitamin B6 50-200 mg per day. The following minerals should be supplemented, at least to RDA - calcium 800-1000 mg, magnesium 300-400 mg, zinc 10-30 mg, chromium 200 mcg, molybdenum 100 mcg, and iodine 200 mcg per day. The dose of iodine should be calculated to body size and need, since overdose is toxic. Pregant women may require carefully calculated increased iodine. We are assuming that the sources of mineral supplements are relatively uncontaminated with radioactive isotopes. Calcium obtained from animal bones or oyster shells will contain environmental contaminants, including isotopes, but calcium obtained from limestone (dolomite) will not be contaminated by recent radioactive fallout.

9.2.8 Carcinogens

Some cancers are caused by specific chemicals. There are at least 350 certified carcinogens producing 80 different tumors In animals and man. Human cancer is known to be produced by at least 130 different chemicals.[36] Radioactive isotopes have already been identified as carcinogenic. Industrial carcinogens include asbestos, benzene, cadmium oxide, chromium, nickel, vinyl chloride, soots, and tars. Several medicinal drugs are carcinogenic. The most potent carcinogenic drugs are those used to treat cancer! Many cancer patients trade remission of today's cancer for the induction of a subsequent cancer in years to come.

Food additives have been closely scrutinized as potential carcinogens, and several, like saccharin, cyclamate, Ponceau 3R, and Red No. 2 (amaranth), have been banned by the FDA because of concern about possible cancer causation. Only one foodborne carcinogen is definitely known, the aflatoxins (produced by aspergillus fungi) contaminating peanuts, wild soy sauce, and grains. It is ironic that foods advocated by some "health food" fans are most likely to be contaminated with aflatoxins. Many other substances are suspected. The surface of the gastrointestinal tract is most intensely exposed to ingested carcinogens. Fortunately, stomach cancer has been declining in the US for many years. Some have suggested that increased vitamin C is responsible, reducing in the formation of nitrosamines. Cancer of the colon, on the other hand, is not declining, and suggests that the late stages of food-processing in the GIT produce a carcinogen. The incidence of colon cancer is positively correlated with the intake of animal food and fat, and negatively correlated with the intake of vegetable foods. Increased vegetable consumption, with inclusion of the Brassica group (cauliflower, cabbage, broccoli, Brussels sprouts) is now recommended. The liver is the most common site beyond the GIT for a foodborne carcinogen to work, since it receives most of the absorbed input from the GIT. The incidence of primary liver cancer is low and declining in the US (0.7%), which does not suggest increasing foodborne carcinogens. Two scholarly reviews of food-related carcinogens are recommended for further reading: Stich's "Carcinogens and Mutagens in the Environment" and Reddy and Cohen's "Diet, Nutrition, and Cancer: A Critical Evaluation".[37,38]

9.2.9 Ill-Defined Illness

The clinical diagnosis of any form of food-related illness always raises the question of food contaminants. The problem is that we never know what role contaminants play, and we have no technology readily available to find out. The postulate that Agent X in the food supply is causing the problem, or promoting the problem, is always viable. The neglect of imponderable factors in our food supply is surely one of the contributors to ignorance about, and denial of, ill-defined illnesses in contemporary populations.

When diet revision works, have we simply removed sufficient quantities of molecular stressors and contaminants to relieve the illness? The answer is unknown. In my city, Vancouver, known for its healthy environment, the summer of 1985 brought clusters of food-related illnesses. The first batch of poisonings was caused by pesticide contamination of greenhouse-grown English cucumbers. Shortly thereafter, another rash of poisoning was blamed on chemically contaminated watermelons from California. In the summer of 1986, we were faced with a measurable increase in radioactive contamination of our food and water. These experiences are duplicated in every city, regularly. Anonymous and accidental contamination of food is augmented by deliberate food sabotage. Threats of cyanide adulteration of grapes led to widespread withdrawal of Chilean fruit in the summer of 1989.

Surveillance may detect chemical contamination before the food reaches consumers, but it is unrealistic to expect that government monitoring alone can assure an uncontaminated food supply. It is also unrealistic to believe official reports that the incidence of contamination-related illness is very low, since the majority of the potential problem is concealed from official view. Systematic population studies, relating illness patterns to food selection, to tissue levels of different environmental contaminants, are needed to assess the prevalence of contaminant illness. An Ontario study, for example, clearly correlated admissions to hospital for respiratory disease with increasing levels of air pollution. Air pollution may not be apparent by taste, smell, color, or transparency. The occurrence of increased respiratory distress in sensitive individuals becomes the most reliable indicator of air pollution. Similarly, contamination of the food supply may not be apparent by taste, smell, color, or texture, but is revealed when increasing numbers of sensitive children become ill.

9.3 Food Protection Policy

Many of the problems in our ecosystem and food supply can only be solved by concerted political action to reduce the growing danger of chemical and radioactive contamination of our environment. I believe that every responsible, thinking citizen should devote time and energy toward the resolution of environmental problems. The 1990's will be the critical decade for us. Either we implicate drastic, effective, environmental protection policies or we will likely suffer increasingly dire consequences in the 21st century. we owe it to our children to fix their local food supply problem and then get to work on the global problems.

A curious property of homo sapiens is that all illness patterns tend to reproduce. A dysphoric population, suffering from food and environmental toxicity, tends to become careless, if not aggressively reckless. A healthy population, feeling vigorous, happy, and well, is more apt to protect its well-being. The path of well-being must begin at the individual level and spiral upward into the rational will of populations intolerant of dysfunction, disease, and suicidal intent.

On an individual level, intelligent selection of food, drink, and environmental conditions may contribute to the resolution of dysfunction, and the maintenance of good health. A workable policy has emerged in the care of sick patients, and may apply to everyone interested in prevention and optimal functioning. The avoidance of most food additives would seem to be a good idea. Additive avoidance falls in the class of general nutritional rules of prevention, joining sodium, sugar, and fat restraint. The avoidance of only specific additives, like food dyes, sulphites, and salicylates, is advocated by some. This avoidance turns into a game, which requires the player to carry rather long lists of foods and food ingredients to stores, where elaborate list-reading and screening procedures are carried out. This is not fun alone. With two or three people, food additive lists can be entertaining, especially if you have prizes for the additive-free product of the day.

The Core Diet policy is less entertaining, more austere, but infinitely more practical. Parents and patients are advised to avoid all manufactured, boxed, bottled, packaged, preserved, and processed food. Packaged and processed meats are given an "X" rating. If this rule is followed, most additives are gone, and the sugar and salt load is dramatically reduced. Shopping strategy is simple - avoid the middle aisles. Most supermarkets place poultry, fish, and produce around the perimeter of the store, and these are the foods we want. You are allowed one or two dashes into the middle isles for toilet paper and soap. You never read labels because you almost never buy labelled food. Frozen vegetables are perfectly acceptable.

The problem of contaminants can be reduced by two simple kitchen procedures - washing and peeling. All fruit and vegetables should be thoroughly washed with clean hot water and a brush, when feasible. If the food has a skin, peel it and throw away the peel. If someone admonishes you, saying that you are throwing away precious nutrients, tell them that it is okay; you are happy to throw out the nutrients with the waxes, dyes, fungicides, pesticides, insect eggs, fungi, radioactive isotopes, bacteria, and viruses. Nutrients are available elsewhere, and proper nutrient accounting will confirm adequate nutrition.

9.3.1 Policy for Cancer Prevention

Cancer prevention begins with modifying children's food supply. The Core Diet path includes features recommended for cancer prevention. The paths of risk factor modification for many illnesses converge toward similar lists of things to do and not to do. This convergence, especially of diet revision policy suggests that a common pathogenesis underlies many different disease processes. The prevention of cancer, high blood pressure, atherosclerosis, diabetes, and senility may all require similar metabolic adjustments, along with the exclusion of molecular stressors, toxins, and carcinogens.

Steps to Reduce Risk of Cancer

> * Maintain a normal body weight
> * Eat poultry and fish – white meat is best
> * Eat from the garden
> * Vegetables supply 60% of daily calories
> * More than 20 grams of fibor content per day
> * Eat Vegetables of the Brassica family
> * Low animal fat, low cholesterol diet
> * Reduce red meat consumption to 1–2 days/week
> * Limit milk intake and dairy products,
> * Do not smoke, charcoal broil, barbecue, or salt-cure
> * Eat only a few eggs per week (3–4)
> * Avoid nitrates, nitrites
> * Avoid other harmful food additives
> * Do not smoke

Be politically active to protect yourself, your children, your world from radioactive isotopes. Nuclear bombs are the largest health risk. The only reason for having nuclear weapons is that we believe we have more enemies than friends. Clearly the task is to make friends with enemies. Nuclear reactors are a problem and nuclear waste promises to haunt us for centuries to come. Do not be easily reassured by "authorities" that everything Is okay. Be involved in nuclear reactor decisions. Get better information, and be intelligently skeptical. While technical optimism is a good thing, Murphy's Law is always true: If something can go wrong, it always will...sooner or later. Healthy optimism is tempered by a realistic sense of our limitations.

Environmental protection standards for air, water, food, and the workplace should be rigorously reviewed, improved, and observed. Take action when chemical exposure occurs at work. Assume that illness patterns related to work environments using chemicals, solvents, cleaning agents, plastics, gases are due to chemical toxicity until proven otherwise. Avoid prolonged exposure to household cleaning fluids, bleach, ammonia, solvents, and paint thinners. Some may be hazardous if inhaled in high concentrations. Pesticides, fungicides, and other home garden and lawn chemicals are also potentially dangerous. Avoid using chemical sprays inside your home.

Glossary Chapters 10 & 11	
BOFA	Beta Oxidation of Fatty Acids
CIC	Circulating Immune Complex
GIT	Gastro–intestinal Tract
Gluten	Wheat Proteins
Ig(A,D,G,E,M)	Immunoglobulins
IME	Inappropriate Molecular Entry
IMED	Inappropriate Molecular Entry Disease

Chapter 10

THE IMMUNE SYSTEM

This chapter introduces the immune system. This is background reading for a better understanding of allergic disease. There are many complicated ways that our food supply interacts with the Immune system. It is best to think of our food supply as a stream of molecular events which the immune system monitors 24 hours a day, every day you live. Sometimes the immune surveillance system is happy and peaceful - all is well. Sometimes the immune system objects to the food stream, and declares, in loud, unpleasant immune language, that all is not well.

10.0.1 Immune System as Defense

The *Immune System* is a distributed network of cells and their molecular products. The principle function of the immune system is defense against infection and invasion of the body space by foreign molecules. The *Immune Defense System* covers all body surfaces exposed to the environment - skin, respiratory tract, gastrointestinal tract, and genitourinary tract. The immune sytem is also distributed in discrete organs of the lymphatic system which includes lymph nodes, tonsils, liver, and spleen. The remainder of the immune system is found circulating in the blood stream or patrolling organ tissues. Some cells of the immune system produce antibodies which identify specific foreign molecules or cell-surface markers. Other immune cells directly attack foreign cells or materials, removing them from the body space. We can think of the immune system as a defending army with many divisions and complicated strategies. Immune defense intends to stop infection and otherwise protect us from invasion by foreign substances. The immune system consists of several populations of cells circulating in our blood stream and patrolling within tissue spaces throughout our body. Another task of the immune system is to detect and destroy abnormal, "strange", and improperly labelled cells. Tissue transplanted into your body will be rejected and destroyed by your immune system because the cells are improperly labelled. Transplant surgery is made possible by matching donor and receptor as closely as possible for the same cell labels. Cell labels are known as histocompatibility antigens or MHC (major histocompatibility complex).

10.0.2 Lymphatic System

The organs of the immune system are collectively called the *"Lymphatic System"*. Everyone has had the experience of lymph nodes swelling during the course of a viral or bacterial infection. Tonsils are part of the lymphatic defense system and are naturally enlarged, particularly in children who are often busy fighting off infections, making new antibodies, and accumulating resistence or immunity to these and related infections. Enlarged tonsils and lymph nodes are just doing their job. The cell populations of the immune system are diverse, but are collectively referred to as *"white blood cells"*. White blood cells are routinely counted and recognized differentially on stained blood smears. The different WBC groups which are readily recognized include lymphocytes, neutrophils, eosinophils, basophils, and monocytes.. These cells are made in the bone marrow and the lymphatic tissues (lymph nodes, thymus, spleen, and gut-associated lymphatic tissue).

10.0.3 Humoral Immunity: Antibodies and Mediators

Our immune system has a cell-defense strategy and a molecular weapon system. Antibodies are proteins made to fit specific molecular shapes, referred to as *antigens*. Antibodies identify foreign antigens and their combination triggers the release or manufacture of mediators which excite a variety of powerful body reactions which are never comfortable and are not always helpful. Antibodies are found circulating in the blood stream, on body surfaces, attached to cell surfaces, and floating in tissue spaces. The antibodies are all proteins and fall into four major groups with different functions. Lymphocytes are the cells which recognize antigens, proliferate after contact with antigens, attack antigen-labelled cells, and manufacture antibodies. These cells belong to many different functional groups which interact in a complex way, resembling a large policing organization. Some T-Lymphocytes (Killer cells or K-cells) act directly to attack cells labelled for attack and are responsible for cell-mediated delayed reactions (Type IV). Some T-lymphocytes act as controllers of the antibody-producing cells, the B-Lymphocytes. Controller T-cells fall into groups which suppress immune response (Suppressor cells) and opposing groups which enhance immune response (Helper cells). We know the system works by delicate checks and balances, and is prone to error. Major error means big trouble for us. B-lymphocytes make antibodies to specific antigens. B-lymphocytes are activated by the helper T-lymphocytes who can remember an antigen once they are sensitized to it.

10.0.4 Inflammation as Immune Reaction

Inflammation is the most powerful effect of immune defense. Inflammation is recognized as *swelling, pain, heat, and redness* in the effected tissue. Inflammation is produced by immune cells within the tissue, releasing specific mediators which control local circulation and cell activities. The ancient purpose of inflammation is to war on invading microorganisms. Inflammation occurs around a skin infection like a boil or may occur within a tendon (tendinitis), a joint (arthritis), or a vital organ. The suffix "...itis" simply means inflammation. Many of the diseases which afflict us are produced by immune-mediated inflammation in target organs. Medical therapy is often directed at controlling inflammation. Apparently nature has provided a good protective strategy in the inflammatory process, but it does go too far too often!

10.0.5 Summary: The Cellular Immune System

Immune cell populations fall into three main groups:

1. Lymphocytes; T-Cells...helpers, supressors, killers. Some lymphocytes transform into plasma cells and make antibodies to specific antigens. Antigen is the molecule which excites antibody production. Antibodies are protein molecules which can capture or bind to specific antigens (like a key fits a lock).

2. B-Cells...antibody-producing cells; become plasma cells when activated to divide and produce antibody.

3. Neutrophils...(polymorphonuclear leukocytes) swallow bacteria and other large invaders.

4. Macrophages...are active in lymphatic tissues (reticuloendothelial system); identify and present the foreign antigen to lymphocytes, beginning the immune defense response.

10.0.6 Summary: The Humoral Immune System

Antibodies are Immunoglobulins (Ig). There are 5 main types.

1.   IgA...secreted on all defended body surfaces – the first defence against invaders.

2.   IgD...an antibody which acts as a receptor on lymphocytes.

3.   IgE...produces typical allergy or immediate hypersensitivity reactions like hay fever, some asthma, hives, and anaphylaxis. Its "normal" function seems to be in antiparasite defence. IgE is measured by a blood test, by skin tests, and by RAST.

4.   IgG...the major circulating antibody which enters tissues freely and participates in diverse immune events.

5.   IgM...the big antibody which mostly defends the blood stream against invading antigens. This antibody likely is the major defense against macromolecules absorbed from the bowel. Its levels are often elevated in the delayed pattern food allergy.

10.0.7 Gastrointestinal Tract Immunity

The surface of the gastrointestinal tract is constantly exposed to antigenic molecules, especially proteins and peptides. It is the largest and most important immunizing surface in our body. Food allergy is a natural consequence of immunity devloped against food antigens. An immunoglobulin, IgA, is secreted on the surface of the gastrointestinal tract as the first line of defence. Immune cells occupy positions within the gastrointestinal tract wall as secondary sentinels. The *mast cell* is an immune cell filled with powerful mediators which it releases if an antigen reacts with antibodies coating its surface. Mast cell mediators, like histamine, serotonin, lymphokines, and bradykinin, are responsible for many of our allergic symptoms.

10.0.8 Reactivity vs. Tolerance

There are specialized areas of the gastrointestinal tract which sample the antigenic material in the GIT fluids. These sampling nodes probably result in the recognition of most food antigens by lymphocytes. Therefore, we are likely "sensitized" to all the food we ingest as a matter of course. The old ideas of "getting allergic to..." some foods and not others are likely misleading. What determines our reactivity is the balance between immune tolerance and immune excitation. This balance is complex. We cannot say why one person begins to react to food and another remains tolerant. The most important consideration is the pattern of food ingestion and its effect on digestion and GIT surface defenses. Any eating pattern which exceeds digestive capacity, or which alters GIT permeability, is likely to result in problems.

10.0.9 Immune Complexes

If an antigen makes its way through the GIT wall, an immune response may result in local inflammation. If antigens make it into the blood stream, *circulating antibodies and immune cells* may react, releasing mediators; or circulating antibodies may attach to the antigen, forming a complex capable of exciting a cascade of dysfunction. This process results in complex delayed immune reactions, which will be described as *Type II, III, and IV allergy* - different from the common atopic or *Type I allergy*. We have realized that peptides (protein fragments) may act as antigens. This means that a person who inadequately digests proteins and absorbs short-chain peptides is very likely to develop an internalized allergy with whole-body consequences. If protein digestion works perfectly, the longest peptide absorbed would have only three or four amino acids linked together. A 4-amino acid peptide would not act as an antigen. A slightly larger amino-acid chain may act as an antigen.

All blood coming from the gastrointestinal tract goes through the liver where most of antigenic macromolecules are removed. If antigens or antigen-antibody complexes pass the liver filter, they may cause disturbances in many organs. Food allergy can only be understood as a *multisystem disorder*. The other path of absorption of molecules from the GIT is through lymphatic drainage. The lymph channels flow together to form the thoracic duct, a flimsy vessel which drains its contents into the subclavian vein. This pathway may direct antigenic molecules directly to the lungs where food antigens may excite asthmatic attacks, bronchitis, or more serious and enigmatic inflammatory lung diseases.

The combination of antibody with antigen in the blood stream is called a circulating immune complex (CIC).

CIC's have the general form of:

Antigen----IgM----Antigen

or

Antigon----IgG

The Core Diet for Kids

CIC's may simply be removed from the circulation by macrophages or they may trigger a cascade of events which lead to multiple symptoms, and possibly tissue damage:

CIC's ---> Mediator release ---> Symptoms

Mediators + Immune cells ---> Inflammation
---> Tissue damage

10.0.10 Failure of Surface Defenses

Many conditions allow antigens access to the body by interfering with GIT-surface defences. Deficiency in the surface IgA antibody defence typically leads to delayed forms of foods allergy. Without adequate IgA, large molecules are routinely absorbed through the gastrointestinal tract wall. Typically a bout of intestinal allergy will develop after a viral infection. Some children are born with defective gastrointestinal tracts or a genetic enzyme deficiency which sets the stage for later problems. Toxic food elements may set up a surface problem. The toxic elements in our environment are usually too complex to define, but must, in some patients, interfere with gastrointestinal tract function and promote the more serious forms of food allergy. Many of my patients find that their food sensitivity varies impressively with changes in their ambient environments. Dysfunction of digestion-supporting organs (liver, pancreas, gall bladder) may also predispose to problems on the surface, permitting access of antigenic macromolecules. Any deficiency in the digestive process may promote the absorption of macromolecules, particularly inadequately digested protein pieces. Allergic responses to food are complex. The simplest classification is to note both immediate and delayed responses. The main task addressed in this workbook is the solution to the more complex and least understood patterns of food intolerance. Consult the following summary for details of the immune reaction types.

10.0.11 Summary of the Food Allergy Complex

Immune responses to food molecules are probably ubiquitous and common causes of human symptoms and disease. The evaluation of food reactivity is difficult and requires a concerted effort of both patient and physician, using a variety of techniques. The commonest error in evaluating allergic phenomena is to assume a static and linear relationship between antigenic stimulus and symptomatic response. Consistency is not a feature of immune responses, especially to ingested antigens where multiple variables of digestion and absorption determine the consequences of eating. The immune system fluxes continuously and rhythmically.

Type I Immediate Hypersensitivity reactions are commonly called "Allergic" and begin as soon as the allergen (antigen) contacts immune cells. The most severe immediate reaction is anaphylaxis, a life-threatening reaction, best known following bee or wasp stings and the ingestion of some foods like nuts, and shellfish.

Type II Cytotoxic reactions are more complex and occur in the blood-stream when antigen gets inside, coats important cells (like red blood cells) which are then attacked by circulating antibody, or humoral "bullets" like complement. A cell so attacked is usually damaged or killed. This sort of reaction can lead to serious problems like hemolytic anemia.

Type III Immune Complex reactions also occur in the blood stream, when antigen gets inside and forms complexes with circulating antibody. These immune complexes may be safely cleared, but are potentially very damaging to us. Immune complexes tend to activate mediator reactions, promote inflammation, and cause organ damage. The classic expression of this illness pattern is "serum sickness" first observed with the injection of animal-derived anit-toxins. Serum sickness is routinely produced by foods, and may present as a serious, life-threatening illness.

Type IV Delayed Hypersensitivity reactions are delayed responses which come on days after a challenge by foreign antigens. This response is mediated by T-lymphocytes and is the basis for skin tests for diseases like tuberculosis. This mechanism is responsible for rejecting foreign cells as in an organ transplant rejection, in blood transfusion reactions, or in the defense against cancer cells which may be identified as foreign and attacked.

Types II, III, IV, and V allergic responses are not obvious and present as chronic complex problems involving many symptoms and many organ systems. The diagnosis is made by history and trials of dietary change monitored by food-diary techniques. Fasting is the quickest method of reducing symptoms, and may be supported by a commercially prepared elemental diet (Tolerex). The treatment of choice is a sustained hypoallergenic diet, custom-fitted to each patient, with avoidance of reactive foods, and with support of digestion and nutrition. Drug therapy with a variety of blocking agents is sometimes desirable.

Type V...I add a fifth category of immune reactivity which represents the disturbance most common in my patients. Type V describes a mixed, sequential pattern of immune response to ingested and absorbed antigens. The most common and severe forms of food allergy are probably Type V mixed immune responses (with Type III reactions leading the way). None of the classical immune processes is likely to occur independent of the other three types of immune injury. For example, when gastrointestinal tract pain and diarrhea are involved in food allergy the sequence is likely to be:

Food ingestion --> partial digestion --> antigen emerges --> antigen meets antibody (IgE) coated mast cells --> mediators released with immediate hypersensitivity symptoms --> increased gastrointestinal tract permeability --> increased absorption of antigenic macromolecule --> CIC's --> systemic mediators released --> multisystem disturbances --> tissue inflammation --> T-lymphocyte activation --> cell-mediated immune response with delayed hypersensitivity reactions.

Dogmatic views of the definition and nature of "Allergy" have prevented some physicians from exploring the many possibilities of dietary therapy that biological insights continue to suggest. The results of thoughtfully directed individualized dietary change are often well worth the effort and expense of achieving them. Remarkable remissions of chronic symptoms are a common reward for the efforts of patients willing to go through major dietary change. The food allergist may be appropriately consulted in the care of patients with complex and serious disorders, especially where symptom complexes suggest a multisystem disorder of unknown origin. The discussion of food allergy in children is continued in the next chapter.

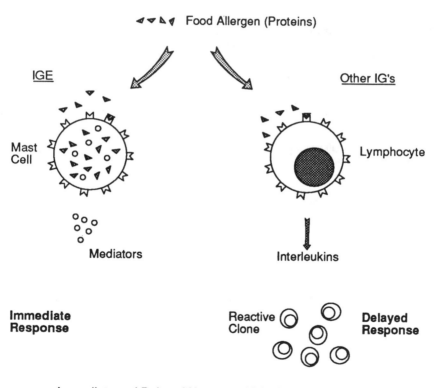

Immediate and Delayed Hypersensitivity Reactions

Chapter 11

FOOD ALLERGY

Our food brings a recurrent stream of molecular traffic and transactions, sense and nonsense, into our body space which has to be sorted out, organized, and cleaned up. The immune defense system acts as a complex military organization, defending against external invasion while maintaining internal law and order. Immune defense must play a major role in screening the traffic in food molecules through the GIT wall, and later in body spaces. Immune defense must recognize the larger, nonsense molecules that leak through the GIT wall, sorting problem food molecules from normal native molecules and disposing of them.

Our only stipulation for the use of the word "allergy" is that the problems so described involve immune responses which disturb or damage in some way. The pattern of illness, the sequence of symptom production, and the distribution of disturbances in the body can be explained if we assume complex causation, including various kinds of immune responses in GIT, blood, and tissue spaces. The timing of sequential immune responses to food can be predicted from basic immunology, and followed clinically by careful recording of symptoms emerging in response to food challenges.

Often a burst of symptoms emerging over hours or days can only be explained if we assume that antigenic material from food has entered the circulation from the GIT and has triggered a variety of alarm and defense procedures.

No specific diagnostic tests define the body's dysfunctional response to food. Spot sampling, so typical of clinical medicine, is seldom helpful in discovering what is wrong. Too often doctors misinform their patients by doing routine spot sample lab tests and then reassuring their patient that "nothing is wrong" when these tests results are normal. This easy reassurance is something like a mechanic checking your tire inflation pressure, and then reassuring you that your car is mechanically sound. Food allergy is diagnosed by physicians who understand the multisystem, polysymptomatic patterns of illness involved. These patterns are revealed by a careful clinical history, and the diagnosis is made on clinical grounds.

11.0.1 Different Patterns of Allergy

The clinical practice of "Allergy" as a specialty has tended to restrict the definition of allergy to one specific pattern of immune reactivity, described as "atopy" by Coca and Cooke in 1925.[39] Specific atopic diseases include hay fever (seasonal allergic rhinitis and conjunctivitis), asthma, eczema, and urticaria (hives). Coca noted several differences between atopic patterns and the life-threatening allergic reaction, anaphylaxis. Anyone could suffer an anaphylactic reaction, but "atopy" tended to occur only in members of predisposed families.

11.0.2 Atopy

Study of the atopic hypersensitivity revealed a more or less definite mechanism which further confirmed the allegiance of many allergists to atopy, with the exclusion of other allergic diseases from their field of interest. It was found that a single antibody species, IgE or "reaginic antibody", was responsible for most of the atopic problems. An atopic allergic reaction is the inflammatory consequences of an allergen meeting an antibody on reactive cell surfaces in various organs - skin, respiratory surfaces, gastrointestinal and genitourinary tracts. For example, an inhaled allergen (antigen), grass pollen, meets antibody-coated mast cells waiting in the mucosal surface of the nose, and a typical hay fever attack with sneezing, itching, and nose congestion results. A similar reaction in the throat produces soreness, mucus flow, swelling, and difficulty in swallowing and breathing (pharyngitis, laryngitis). The same reaction in the lungs produces cough, mucus obstruction to airflow, and asthmatic wheezing (bronchitis, asthmatic bronchitis).

The mast cell is an immune cell filled with powerful mediators which are released if an antigen reacts with antibodies coating the cell's surface. The antibodies are of the IgE type. The tendency to make excessive amounts of IgE antibody is the characteristic of atopic individuals. This tendency is inherited. The reactive surfaces of an atopic individual suffer inflammatory derangement when challenged by incoming antigen. The IgE on the mast cell surface act as triggers when a sufficient number of allergenic molecules are bound to them. When the mast cell is triggered, it releases packets of chemical mediators which cause the allergic symptoms..

A convenient correlation between nose-reactive IgE and skin-reactive IgE was discovered. By injecting tiny amounts of suspected antigens into the skin, a local wheal and flare reaction, like a mosquito bite, is produced if reactive IgE is present on skin mast cells. The association of hay fever, asthma, and skin tests with allergy practice was further confirmed by the relative success of "allergy shots". These shots came to so characterize the allergist's office that other potential aspects of allergy practice often were neglected. Allergy shots, or desensitization, are immunological treatments. They are also referred to as "Immunotherapy". The immune response to any reactive substance can be modified by giving repeated challenges of the reactive substances. Allergy shots for hay fever start with a serum containing the antigens which caused positive skin responses. The antigens are then administered in increasing concentrations by regular injections under the skin. It remains somewhat unclear how the shots work. One response to the injected antigen is the production of a second antibody population of the IgG class. These IgG antibodies are thought to compete with IgE antibodies, "blocking" the allergic response. It is also possible that the antigen injections stimulate supressor T-cells or inhibit helper T-cells and reduce production of IgE.

Allergy shots have limited therapeutic application. The hay fever sufferer and some asthmatics with specific inhalant reactions to grass pollens do well with desensitization.[40] Immunotherapy also protects patients who have had anaphylatic reactions to bee and wasp stings. Patients with complex reactivity, food reactions, and drug reactions do not do well with allergy shots, and the shots are not usually recommended. There are dangers with allergy shots including life-threatening anaphylaxis, delayed immune responses associated with generalized symptoms, and, rarely, a grave illness like polyarteritis nodosa. Indeed the delayed reactions to allergy shots are typical of the immune-mediated disease process which is characteristic of food allergy. It is my policy to avoid allergy shots in patients who have food allergy and other forms of delayed immune responses.

The reason for the definition of "allergy" to shrink toward a narrowly-defined clinical practice probably was the skin test. If anything distinguished an allergist from his medical colleagues, it was the allergist's passion for skin tests. Some still think that an allergist without skin tests is no allergist at all.

By a practical evolution of allergy practice, those clinical problems which were diagnosable by skin reactions became the special property of allergists. Allergy therapy became synonymous with the desensitization (immunotherapy) injections.

11.0.3 Immediate-Reacting Food Allergens

For some time, it has been appreciated that food allergy operates in a more complex and mysterious way than inhaled allergy. Although skin tests were used to test for food sensitivity, many allergists also prescribed food elimination diets on clinical grounds with satisfactory clinical results. Allergists generally appreciated that allergy shots containing food antigens were not helpful. The IgE model was nevertheless the easiest route to follow in the study of food allergy. This model encourages us to search for specific food allergens and to trace the occurrence of similar allergic substances in related foods. An allergic reaction to peanuts, for example, suggests that the peanut protein sensitizer may appear in related legumes like peas or soybeans. This "cross-reactivity" has been noted for several food groups - legumes, citrus fruits, crustaceans, grains, mustards, and so on.

The study of food allergens has focused on the special allergens which produce immediate allergic reactions. A profile of allergenic proteins suggests that glycoproteins of a certain size and weight are common allergens. These proteins can be isolated from foods and are used to skin test sensitive individuals. Specific protein allergens have been characterized from a variety of foods, particularly cow's milk, eggs, soybeans, peanuts, fish, crustaceans, wheat, oats, corn, rice, citrus, and some other foods. Laboratory studies of the interaction of these specific proteins and antibodies present in the blood of sensitive individuals have confirmed the immediate hypersensitivity model of allergy as a reaction between specific proteins and specific antibodies. This model of allergy is immensely satisfying to researchers, because of its simplicity and the ease of testing for sensitization.

The immediate hypersensitivity concept of food allergy selects only a special population of people who show a sensitization to food caused by a single antibody type, IgE. While this is an important reaction pattern, some physicians have claimed it is the only valid form of allergic reactions to food. Their opinion is no longer acceptable.

11.0.4 Inappropriate Molecular Entry Disease

To understand the broader definition of food allergy, our focus is on the interface between things ingested and the inner body space. The boundary is the tubular wall of the GIT. This boundary selects molecules for entry into the private space of self. Understanding the error potential of this boundary is critical to the new understanding of food-related dysfunction and disease.[41,42,43,44] Drs. Coombs and McLaughlin summarized the problem simply in a 1984 discussion of Food Allergens.[45]

> "Food proteins in the gastrointestinal tract and their absorption into the body as antigenic molecules have immunologic significance both in (i) initiating an allergic state and (ii) in the subsequent challenge(s) where, by a variety of mechanisms, they may cause some form of "food-allergic disease".

In nutritional programming language, the wrong absorption of large molecules, especially proteins, is described as "Inappropriate Molecular Entry" (IME). The diseases caused by this mechanism are now called "IMED" - Inappropriate Molecular Entry Disease. The various patterns of food allergy can now be more accurately desribed as patterns of IMED.

Food allergic responses, initiated by the absorption of non-nutrient molecules, typically involve a symptom complex. The multisymptom process begins to make sense when one considers the progression of events from the GIT, to blood stream, to mediators released, to whole-body responses, to long term consequences of inflammatory tissue events, which, once set in motion, tend to persevere. A simple classification of food allergy symptom patterns is based on the timing of symptoms:

The *immediate* responses are symptoms emerging in 1-60 minutes. As the allergy process unfolds, at least two other time periods are readily recognized.

Symptoms like headache, drowsiness, dizziness, cognitive dysfunction, and aching tend to arrive 1-6 hours after eating, and may be classed *intermediate.*

Delayed symptoms emerge in 6-72 hours after eating. Delayed responses may reflect transit and processing time in the intestinal tract. It may, for example, take a food problem 12-48 hours to reach the colon and produce pain and diarrhea, or rectal itching and hemorrhoidal swelling. Many of the inflammatory consequences of food allergy are delayed many hours, emerging slowly and insidiously. It is not possible to think simplistically about immune reactions to food, and understand them.

11.0.5 Inflammation

Inflammation is the most potent effect of immune defense. Inflammation is recognized as swelling, pain, heat, and redness in the affected tissue. Inflammation is produced by immune cells within the tissue, releasing specific mediators which control local circulation and cell activities. The ancient purpose of inflammation is to war on invading microorganisms. Thus, inflammation describes a battle-ravaged tissue.

Inflammation occurs around a skin infection like a boil, or may occur within a tendon (tendinitis), a joint (arthritis) or a vital organ. The suffix "itis" simple means inflammation. Much of the disease which afflicts us is felt as the symptoms of inflammation. Medical therapy is often directed at controlling inflammation. Apparently, nature has provided a good protective strategy in the inflammatory process, but it goes too far too often! The pathologist recognizes different stages and patterns of inflammation from acute to chronic. Under the microscope, an inflamed tissue is invaded by many different cells of the immune system. Many of the chronic and unsolved diseases which plague our civilization are inflammatory disorders. Some of the disorders involve daily suffering, but little tissue damage. The common painful syndrome of fibrositis, otherwise know as the "muscle-fascia syndrome" or "fibromyositis", is an example of a disease involving daily suffering with little to show for it. Children with "growing pains" actually have fibrositis or mild arthritis. Other diseases combine suffering with aggressive destruction of tissue during the inflammatory process. Rheumatoid arthritis is an example of destructive joint inflammation.

11.1 Milk Allergies

The allergy to cow's milk is the best studied food allergy.[46,47,48,49] In the following discussion of cow's milk allergy, the milk proteins serve as a model of all allergenic proteins. The milk proteins can be replaced by beef, pork, egg, soya, peanuts, wheat, oats, rye, barley, corn, potato, peanut, fish, and so on as the mechanisms of food allergic disease are described and the resultant diseases are defined. Once again, it is important to realize that the symptoms of food allergy are prolific and profuse.

11.1.1 Antigens in Milk

Cow's milk contains many proteins which are antigenic. Infants and any adult with gastrointestinal tract disease may have difficulty digesting these proteins and may absorb them as antigens. Casein is the best known milk protein; lactalbumin, lactoglobulin, bovine albumin, and gamma globulin are other protein groups within the milk. There are at least 20 antigenic proteins in milk. Digestion probably increases the number of possible antigens to over 100.

Evidence that digested fractions of each of the milk proteins may induce IgE, IgA, and IgG antibodies suggests variable immune response after eating food combinations. A very good argument can be made that the success and extent of digestion of any given protein will vary over a large range, depending upon multiple factors which govern and control digestion. Complete breakdown of a protein into individual amino acids or peptides consisting of no more than 3 or 4 amino acids will prevent an immunological response to a food. Incomplete digestion of a protein into larger antigenic fragments would encourage an immune response, producing symptoms after eating. The symptom response is variable and emerges from minutes to hours after eating food containing milk proteins. The variability of symptom production can confuse both parents and physicians.

11.1.2 Role of Secretory IgA

The role of the secretory antibody IgA is well studied in milk allergy. This antibody is secreted on the surface of intestinal cells. The role of IgA seems to be to trap undesirable molecules and block their entry into the absorbing surface of GIT. Deficiency of IgA would permit the entry of more allergenic macromolecules into body space via the systemic circulation. Newborn infants are deficient in both serum and secretory IgA. IgA levels rise progressively in a normal child to an adult range over the first four years. This IgA deficiency makes infants more susceptible to food allergy.

IgA deficiency continues in some people as an isolated abnormality, perpetuating a proclivity to food allergy. One of my patients with serum IgA deficiency is an otherwise healthy teenage girl who suffers from episodic attacks of swelling and excessive sleep, suggestive of narcolepsy. She must avoid milk proteins to remain awake and alert. Her symptoms also occur in children with normal IgA, but perhaps not so dramatically.

11.1.3 Incidence of Cow's Milk Allergy

The incidence of cows' milk protein allergy (CMPA) has been estimated according to the immediate hypersensitivity model of allergy to be up to 7% in infants and children. Among atopic children, the estimated incidence of milk allergy is 14-30%. These estimates are based on small, totally inadequate studies, using restricted definitions of "allergy". I believe the incidence of milk allergy is much higher - probably greater than 30% of all children, and as high as 50% in adolescents and adults, if we include all the possible combinations of immune response in the definition of "allergy". Cow's milk is the most common food allergen in childrens' diets. The adult patterns of CMPA are predominantly of the delayed type and present as chronic, complex illness patterns.

11.1.4 Symptoms of Milk Allergy

In infants and children, the many patterns of milk allergy illustrate well that food allergy is a chronic, polysymptomatic, multisystem disorder. The most obvious presentation of milk allergy is the irritable, unhappy infant with regurgitation, vomiting, chronic diarrhea, bouts of colic, scalded buttocks, cheek eczema, and failure to thrive. Eczema is a common presentation of milk allergy in infants and should suggest food allergy until proven otherwise.

Vomiting is the most conspicuous sign of milk allergy. Since infants may be sensitized in utero to cow's milk protein, they may begin vomiting with the first feeding of cow's milk. They may also vomit with breast milk if the mother continues to ingest cow's milk protein. In the newborn, vomiting is alarming and, if it persists, is life threatening. The attending physician must consider a differential diagnosis of vomiting which includes pyloric stenosis, other gastrointestinal tract obstructions, and metabolic disorders, especially the inborn errors of amino acid metabolism. The integrity of the GIT is checked by barium swallow X-rays, and ultrasound. Metabolism is checked by measuring blood chemistry, especially the levels of ammonia, pH, and serum amino acids. The urine is checked for protein and ketones. Cow's milk allergy should be the first diagnosis, revised only if distinct abnormalities are found in the GIT or metabolism.

If her infant has been vomiting for some time, the mother feels frightened, frustrated, and guilty. If the mother is breast feeding, she should follow a hypoallergenic diet with nutrient supplements and should be encouraged to continue breast feeding. She often needs reassurance, guidance, and support, preferably from another nursing mother who has resolved a similar problem. If attempted breast feeding fails, the search for an acceptable alternative begins. The alternatives are described below. If the milk allergy problem is not diagnosed, the mother and infant are candidates for chronic illness, confusion, and despair. The infant continues to vomit, fails to thrive, and may show growth and maturation arrest as long as the food allergy problem remains unresolved. I have witnessed too many examples of this failed diagnosis and the misery of mother and child. Often, in the unresolved situation, the mother is blamed for the feeding failure and may be punished both covertly and overtly by all observers, including physicians and nurses who do not appreciate the profundity of the food allergy problem. The diagnosis of food allergy in infants is made clinically, not by skin tests, nor RAST, and is confirmed when the offending foods are eliminated and improvement occurs. No one should be in any rush to reintroduce allergenic foods.

Diarrhea and malabsorption caused by milk ingestion may be associated with deterioration of the gastrointestinal tract surface, which impairs digestion and absorption of other food molecules. Any food allergy which disturbs gastrointestinal tract function tends to multiply its effects. This is why a major comprehensive dietary change is often necessary to resolve a food-intolerance problem. Milk allergy tends to produce gluten intolerance, for example, and visa versa.

Other infants and children present with less obvious gastrointestinal effects, but more evident effects in their respiratory tract (nasal congestion, excess throat mucus, middle ear fluid, cough, croup, bronchitis). The infant respiratory syndrome tends to peak at 4-12 months and may not be suspected as the cause of frequent "colds" or "bronchitis". These children are chronically congested, cough recurrently, and sometimes have asthmatic wheezing. Many children with milk and other food allergy have recurrent ear "infections" and are treated inappropriately with repeated courses of antibiotics or decongestants, and often have tubes inserted through their ear drums. The diagnosis of food allergy is seldom considered, but must be the most frequent cause of this common problem. Permanent hearing loss may result from this neglect and too many children have hearing-impaired learning disability from this correctable cause.

Occasionally, milk allergy presents as anemia, secondary to blood loss from a milk-inflamed gastrointestinal tract and/or malabsorption of essential blood-forming nutrients (especially iron). These milk allergy patterns are not dependent on the IgE mechanism and cannot be diagnosed by allergy skin tests. The diagnosis is made clinically and is proven by good results on a hypoallergenic diet.

Behavioral effects of milk allergy manifest the interaction of peptides and/or immunologic mediators with the infant brain causing behavioral disturbances such as irritability, excessive crying or screaming, insomnia, hyperactivity, or, paradoxically, listlessness and apathy. In infants and older children, the behavioral effects include irritability, temper tantrums, restless sleep, and clumsiness or uncoordination. Later, in school, these children show attention deficits and often are thought to have learning disabilities. The behavioral disturbance syndrome can occur with any food allergy - milk is simply a common culprit.

Skin eruptions vary from common eczema to measles-like rashes and hives. The cheeks and/or ears of allergic infants and children typically are brightly flushed following ingestion of milk or similar allergens. Itching and squirming behavior are associated with flushing in the acute allergic reactions.

In older children and adults, the pattern of reaction tends to change. Indigestion manifested as heartburn, excessive gas, and crampy abdominal pain are common symptoms. Respiratory symptoms - chronic nose congestion, cough, and, sometimes, asthma - remain a problem. The appearance of leg pain is common in 3-4 year olds who now can describe their symptoms. These "growing pains" are typical of mast cell mediator release in connective tissues. The unlucky child will develop a serious inflammatory arthritis which looks like rheumatic fever or rheumatoid arthritis. Again, the correct diagnosis of food allergy is often not made and these children receive the most inappropriate, and sometimes dangerous, treatment. Skin tests are not helpful.

Curious brain effects are described by adult patients; these include excessive sleepiness, aching, restless legs, burning sensations deep inside arms and legs, and a generalized restlessness which may be dramatically disturbing. Infants and children cannot describe these disturbances well, but show their distress in disturbed behavior or fitful sleep as they experience similar sensations.

11.1.5 Time Sequences

The onset and duration of milk allergy, like any other food allergy is confusingly variable. In infants, symptoms of milk intolerance may begin immediately or within a month of milk ingestion. After a milk feeding, typical symptoms may begin in a few minutes as acute hypersensitivity, but other symptoms may be delayed as long as 1-3 days (17% of symptoms were delayed according to one study). There is a tendency for the immediate milk sensitivity reactions (IMD.E1) in young infants to diminish as they get older. Half of infants afflicted in the first year may show "milk tolerance" after one year. The best understanding of milk and food allergy is, however, that the problem may come and go at any age, is likely to be variable, and is likely to change in severity and symptom production over observation periods of many years. The delayed patterns of food allergy are likely to appear after the immediate sensitivity has abated.[50] The infant with milk-induced vomiting and diarrhea from 4-14 months may seem to tolerate the reintroduction of milk at 14 months, but, months or years later will develop eczema, fatigue, abdominal pain, "growing pains", and the chronic respiratory syndrome, with cough, wheezing, and nose congestion. Or these children may simply have attention deficit disorder with learning and behavioral problems. The early symptoms vanish as the food allergy patterns change with growth, changing eating habits, and changing environments.

After a trial of milk elimination, reintroduction of milk products may not reproduce symptoms immediately. Respiratory symptoms, in particular, may take several days to three weeks to reappear.[51]

11.1.6 Treatment of Milk Allergy

Elimination of milk and milk products is the essential treatment for anyone with milk allergy. Further diet modification is often necessary because food allergy is often a non-specific disease, involving many different foods. In managing delayed patterns of food allergy, one must be prepared to restrict cereal grain gluten, eggs, some meats, often soya protein, some fruits (especially citrus), sugars, and food additives. The Core Diet approach advocated in this book should be utilized whenever the problem is more complex than a simple single food intolerance.

Substitutes for cows' milk include goat's milk and milk products manufactured from soya beans. Goat's milk may also cause allergic responses and is often expensive or difficult to obtain. It is common practice to utilize a commercially-prepared hydrolysed soy protein formula containing carefully balanced nutrients (Isomil, Soyalac, Prosobee, Nursoy). Regular soy milk should not be used to feed infants. Soy milk is not an ideal food for infants and requires considerable modification before it is nutritionally competent and safe for infants. Even carefully thought-out infant soy formulas may be deficient in subtle ways. The Wyeth company (manufacturer of Nursoy), for example, recently modified their formula by adding L-carnitine. They appreciated that L-carnitine is supplied in breast and cow's milk, but is not available in vegetable foods like soya. Carnitine is essential for the proper utilization of fatty acids in BOFA. In the first few months of life, infants may not produce enough carnitine to run BOFA at peak efficiency. Nursoy now has 7 mg of carnitine per litre of formula.[52] The infant soy formulas can also be useful for older children and adults who do not tolerate cow's milk. The soy formula can be used in place of canned milk in cooking, or as a complete nutritional supplement when food choices are limited.

It is important to realize that soy protein allergy is also common and the soy milk formulas may produce as much disturbance as cow's milk formulas. The incidence of soya allergy is about one third that of cow's milk; 40% of infants allergic to cow's milk also show adverse reactions to soy milk formulas, although the onset may be delayed several weeks. For infants and adults with cow's milk and soy formula intolerance, partially hydrolysed protein "hypoallergenic formulas" may be used. These include Nutramigen and Pregestimil. These are Mead Johnson products supplying protein as an enzymatic hydrosylate of casein, the milk protein with the least allergenic potential. Pregestimil also contains individual amino acids and the fat is presented as medium-chain triglycerides, desirable when gastrointestinal tract absorption is impaired. Recently, another hypoallergenic milk product has been announced by Carnation. They have produced an infant formula, "Good Start HA", with hydrolysed whey, and claim better results in both treating and preventing food allergy in susceptable infants. Unfortunately the hydrolysis of milk proteins leaves allergenic possibilities - some infants are likely to have problems with any hydrolysed protein product. For non-breast-fed infants who do not tolerate soy protein and hydrolysed protein formulas, an elemental formula may be the only safe nutrient supply. Knowledgeable physician supervision is essential.

In summary, the infant feeding path is a progression of choices. When infant problems occur, the feeding choices are modified progressively until the problem is resolved:

1. Breast milk. Modify mother's diet if problems are encountered.
2. If mother cannot feed, consider a human milk donor.
3. If not breast milk, and if problems, then:
4. Infant soya milk formula. If problems, then:
5. Hypoallergenic formula, Nutramigen. If problems, then:
6. Hypoallergenic formula, Pregestimil. If problems, then:
7. Elemental nutrient formula.

11.1.7 Lactose Intolerance

Milk allergy may be imitated in its gastrointestinal tract consequences by a milk sugar digestive abnormality. The milk sugar, lactose, is a dissacharide which requires a specific enzyme, lactase, to be digested into its two component sugars, glucose and galactose. When the activity of lactase is insufficient to digest the lactose presented to the GIT, lactose is not absorbed and passes through the GIT into the colon. Colon bacteria ferment the undigested lactose, producing abundant gas and lactic acid. This fermentation feels very uncomfortable and may result in GIT inflammation with diarrhea.

Milk lactose in the GIT of lactase-deficient patients seems to interfere with calcium absorption; 18% reduction in calcium absorption has been reported. Yogurt is relatively free of lactose and is a good source of calcium for lactase deficient patients who tolerate milk proteins.

Lactase deficiency may be inherited or may develop during the course of many gastrointestinal tract diseases. Ingesting milk may aggravate or prolong the course of any diarrheal illness. Tablets containing lactase may be ingested along with milk products to compensate for intrinsic enzyme deficiencies, although milk restriction is usually a more satisfactory course of action. Lactase (Lactaid) is of no benefit to milk allergy. Soy milk products contain no lactose and are suitable substitutes for cow's milk when soy protein is tolerated.

11.1.8 Galactose & Metabolic Food Intolerance

Milk produces dysfunction and disease in other ways. Some infants are born with a deficiency of an enzyme which converts galactose to glucose (galactose-1-phosphate uridyl transferase). Galactose accumulates in their bodies when they are fed milk and it poisons them. They develop diarrhea, colic, liver enlargement, and cataracts, and, if untreated, they suffer damage to their growing brains, producing mental retardation. These infants must not drink milk if they are to be spared major damage, since the lactose contributes galactose which they cannot metabolize. Soy milk also contains galactose and is not permitted in galactose intolerance. Galactose intolerance illustrates the general class of metabolic problems produced by enzyme deficiencies, blocking the metabolism of specific nutrient molecules which accumulate and cause disease. It should be recognized that enzyme deficiencies need not be completely expressed, as in the case of infants with galactosemia, but may be partial and intermittent and may come on at any age.

11.2 Cereal Grains and Disease

Foods made with milk and wheat are the staples in the North American and European diets. Wheat and its close relatives, oats, barley, and rye, have proved to be major problems in the diets of sick children. One of the most awkward and undesirable features of the Core Diet is the complete exclusion of the cereal grains. A brief review of some of the reasons for excluding these popular foods follows.

11.2.1 Cereal Grain Intolerance

The nutritional benefits of grains may cost too much in terms of dysfunction and disease. Some of us must avoid whole grains totally to remain well, and others must moderate their intake to improve digestion and absorption of essential nutrients. Craving and compulsive eating of flour-based foods is common, especially the reward and dessert foods containing sugar. Some have difficulty digesting increased grains and suffer GIT disturbances. Others have allergic or idiosyncratic reactions to the grain proteins and suffer a generalized illness. Others have brain dysfunction - sleepiness, attention deficits, and depression. Others develop skin disease, connective tissue inflammation, and arthritis. Whole grains also contain phytates which bind desirable minerals, preventing their absorption. Calcium, magnesium, and zinc deficiencies may occur with diets high in whole grains.

The clinical presentations of cereal-grain intolerance include:

* Lethargy, fatigue, sleepiness, and insomnia
* Diarrhea, chronic, with malabsorption, weight loss, micronutrient deficiencies, blood loss, and anemia
* Abdominal pain, recurrent and associated with increased gas and distention
* Anemia may be the presenting problem with associated abdominal pain and distension. Anemia results from malabsorption of one or more nutrients essential to blood formation – iron, folic acid, and Vitamin B12
* Skin Disorders – acne-like skin eruptions, eczema, dermatitis herpetiformis
* Respiratory Disease – rhinitis, bronchitis, and asthma
* Aching, stiffness, leg pains
* Arthritis
* Brain dysfunction esp attention deficts, depression
* Schizophrenia?

11.2.2 The Gluten Proteins

Wheat proteins are collectively called "Gluten". Wheat is closely related to other cereal grains, especially rye, barley, and oats. There has been a renewed enthusiasm for "whole grains" and increased dietary fiber, especially in the past decade, leading to increased consumption of these cereals in a relatively unrefined form and often in combination, as with granola cereals and whole wheat breads fortified with bran, coarse flours, and other additives. Gluten is a mixture of individual proteins classified in two groups, the Prolamines and the Glutelins. The prolamine fraction of gluten concerns us the most when grain intolerance is suspected. The most troublesome component of gluten is the prolamine, Gliadin. Gliadin in wheat seems to be the major problem in celiac disease, and gliadin antibodies are most commonly found in the immune complexes associated with major disease.[53,54] We eat the seeds of the grain plants. The seed has a bran casing, a starchy endosperm which contains 90% of the protein, and a small germ nucleus which is the plant embryo waiting to grow. Any flour made from the starchy endosperm contains prolamines and is potentially toxic to the grain intolerant person.

The disease most often associated with cereal grains or "Gluten intolerance" is the digestive disorder "Celiac Disease", the prototype of wheat allergic disease. When wheat is the principle problem food, there is a concensus that barley, oats, and rye must be excluded as well. Millet is intermediate in the list of offenders. Rice is usually tolerated when gluten prolamines are the chief and only food intolerance. Triticale is a new hybrid grain with the properties of wheat and rye, and is excluded on a gluten-free diet.[55]

11.3 Summary of Food Allergy

In review, the concepts important to our practical understanding of food allergy are:

1. Most foods contain molecules which can act as antigens and excite immune responses. Most, if not all, of us have made antibodies against food components. The response to food is complex and variable, never consistent.

2. An interactive, often synergistic effect of molecular stressors in air, food, water, and drugs should be predicted and taken into account.

3. The gastrointestinal tract does not always process food well, and may permit the absorption of antigenic large molecules quite routinely. The absorption of intact proteins likely occurs in most people on a regular basis. Gastrointestinal tract function changes progressively throughout life, and is especially vulnerable to toxic stressors common in our diets, to interference by infections, and to iatrogenic disturbances from surgery, hospital procedures, ill-conceived diets, and too many drugs, especially antibiotics.

4. In people with the most serious form of food allergy, the GIT is excessively permeable and macromolecular absorption occurs on a regular and intense basis. The pattern of multisystem disorder in patients with food allergy is better understood as a consequence of Inappropriate Molecular Entry (IME). The admission of antigenic food molecules into the body can initiate complicated patterns of immune-mediated disease (IMD).

5. The patterns of illness are determined by sequences of immune mechanism, triggered by the presence of aberrant molecules in the circulation and/or tissue spaces. These patterns have not yet been adequately described and may underlie many of the common, serious, and unexplained diseases.

6. The distinction between immediate and obvious allergic reactions to food and the delayed, complicated, less obvious immune responses remains clinically useful. Only the immediate reactions are studied and treated in the manner of hay fever-type allergy. The remaining, more profound problems of food allergy require sophisticated approaches to define, understand, and resolve the disease.

Glossary Chapters 12, 13 & 14

ADD	Attention Deficit Disorder
ADHD	Attention Deficit Hyperactivity Disorder
ARF	Adverse Reactions to Foods
BBB	Blood Brain Barrier
CIC	Circulating Immune Complexes
DRT	Diet Revision Therapy
ELIZA	Antibody test
EXM	Expectancy Modes
FAST	Antibody test
ID	Intradermal
Ig(A,G,E,M)	Immunoglobulins
IMED	Inappropriate Molecular Entry Disease
LD	Learning Disabilities
LL1	First Law of Libido
LL2	Second Law of Libido
MAO	Monoamine Oxidase
NE	Norepinephrine
PsyE	Psychic Energy
RAST	Antibody Test
RCL	Recursive Loops
RCLI	Recursive Loop Inducers

Chapter 12

TESTS AND TREATMENTS

The idea of a simple office "test" for food allergy should seem unlikely. The problem is too profound and too complex to ever be evaluated by a simple test. The Core Diet is actually a diagnostic program at the same time as it is a treatment program. The diagnosis of food allergy is confirmed by remission of symptoms on the Core Diet, and is further confirmed by return of symptoms after offending foods are eaten. The desire for simple, definitive tests for food allergy is easy to understand, but difficult to fulfill. A quick review of proposed tests follows.

12.0.1 Allergy Skin Tests

The familiar allergy skin tests, with protein extracts from foods, have proven disappointing and often misleading. The food scratch test still survives because it does reveal the IgE sensitization to foods in people who react this way. The food scratch test does an enormous disservice if it is used to deny food allergy. A negative skin test for food is meaningless. The entire spectrum of delayed pattern food allergy lies beyond the predictive abilities of this elementary form of immunological testing.

12.0.2 Provocation Tests: Sublingual

A group of environmentally aware physicians, known as clinical ecologists, developed "provocation tests for food sensitivity". They wanted to simulate, in a convenient and quick way, the responses of a patient to eating the food. The sublingual provocation test (SLPT) was invented as an office procedure. Dropping the allergenic extract of food under the tongue was an obvious sort of simulation to try. The idea is that some of the food antigens would be absorbed through the mouth lining, and would interact with immune sensors and reactors in the blood. The SLPT simulation would perhaps detect the immediate type responses of circulating basophils. The problem with the SLPT is that it is completely unreliable. The test responses are subjective, the absorption of the antigen under the tongue is variable and unknown, the responses to small doses of antigen are not representative of the illness problem...the list goes on. The SLPT is not diagnostic of food allergy.

12.0.3 Provocation Tests: by Injection

Provocation tests by needle injection of food proteins into the skin have also been used. The intradermal (ID) injections test has proven to be more effective in showing IgG4 reactivity to antigens, and will occasionally show a delayed, cell-mediated response in 48 hours. Again, symptoms may develop as injected antigen reacts with skin mast cells, or reaches circulating basophils and triggers an amplified immediate alarm response. Injected antigen can cause a dangerous anaphylactic response by the mast cell-basophil mechanism. There is no question that injected antigen can cause dramatic symptoms, illustrating one of the mechanisms producing symptoms in the allergic patient. The symptomatic response is not consistent enough, however, to be a reliable test of food allergy. The antigen dose is too small to simulate any of the IMED mechanisms. The ID provocation test is, therefore, no more useful than scratch tests or sublingual tests.

12.0.4 Cytotoxic Tests

Another laboratory test has been offered as the definitive test for "food sensitivity", and subsequently was condemned by the American College of Allergists as ineffective. The idea behind cytotoxic tests has a validity which the commercially applied technique failed to deliver. The second mechanism of immune-mediated disease is the cell-damaging or cytotoxic effect of antigen-antibody interactions. Cells may also be damaged by direct toxicity of drugs and food-related chemicals. The cytotoxic tests, recently marketed, expose blood cells to food extracts in a chamber viewed through a microscope. Automation has been applied to cell counting and evaluation, to produce automated test results. There are many problems with this technique that rob it of practical utility. The question "What is the test simulating?" must be asked of every proposed food allergy test. The major phenomena of food allergy are not cytotoxic effects, although this damage does occur; therefore, the test misses the majority of the problem. If the cytotoxic effect is to be evaluated, does this test do a credible job?

No, it does not. Cells in a salt solution in a counting chamber are sensitive to non-specific physical factors, like light and temperature. Cells may be destroyed by raising or lowering the concentration, or by the pH of the suspending solution. Are the testing substances representative of the food? After eating the food, will blood cells be exposed to the test substances in an identical manner? Cytotoxic tests fail this sort of examination. The idea of developing a valid test of cell response remains viable and deserves more work. The practical point is to save the several hundred dollars usually demanded for cytotoxic testing and to spend it on good hypoallergenic food.

12.0.5 Laboratory Tests

The IgE model of allergy inspired development of antibody-measuring laboratory tests. The idea was to show the affinity of circulating antibodies to different antigens. The hay-fever model dominated test ideas; if you had enough IgE directed to June grass pollen, you would sneeze when you inhaled the pollen. The same reasoning was applied to food allergy, and RAST testing was developed to detect IgE antibodies to different food proteins. For a brief time, the RAST was used instead of, or in addition to, skin scratch tests to attempt the diagnosis of food allergy. Whenever IgE mechanisms dominate the food allergy problem, RAST is a useful test. Variations of the RAST idea allow for antigen-specific antibodies to be assayed. The related tests bear the acronyms ELIZA, FAST, and MAST, and others will appear as this testing technology develops. Negative RAST results were again used to deny food allergy as an explanation of patients' illnesses, and seemed to carry more weight, looking more official and "scientific" on a computer printout from the lab. The IgE response is not the problem in the majority of food allergy cases that I treat; the multiple immune responses to IMED are the major problem. Therefore, IgE RAST is never adequate to diagnose the complexities of food allergy.

The principles of RAST testing for IgE are now applied to the measurement of other antibody types. The measurement of IgG is of great interest. Current studies show frequent IgG responses to food antigens, and reactivity patterns activated by IgG. Recently, new lab tests measuring food-antigen specific IgG have been offered in an impressive computer-reported format.[56] The foods attacked by IgG are listed, and avoidance of these food is advised. Helpful food lists and food rotation instructions accompany the reports. Often, the test results are very specific (you "react to" parmesan cheese, but not to Swiss cheese). The results of this evaluation are so convenient, so professional looking, it would appear the problem of food allergy diagnosis is solved. What are the problems with this approach? Again, we are not sure what the IgG antibodies to food antigens are doing and, therefore, we do not know what reactivity the test simulates. There is little experience in applying the test results clinically, so we do not know if the results of avoiding IgG reactive foods are effective. In my limited experience with the IgG test, the clinical results are not very successful. It is easy to postulate, for example, that the presence of IgG to a food antigen protects you to some extent from the allergic reaction. In pollen allergy, IgG antibodies are thought to block the allergic response mediated by IgE. It may be that we should eat the IgG positive foods and avoid all the others - this is an unlikely postulate, but illustrates our lack of knowledge of the proper application of these lab results.

Evaluation of IgA and IgM antibodies to food antigens is also of great interest. Studies relating levels of all antibody types to clinical observations are needed before the complexities of food allergy will become apparent. No single antibody measurement will predict the immune response to food. No single lab measurement should be used as a diagnostic test for food allergy.

The measurement of total blood levels of four antibody species (immunoglobin electrophoresis) is of some interest in the complex food allergy patterns. Very often, shifts in the distribution of IgG, IgM, IgA, and IgE manifest immune activity in response to antigen loading through GIT. The commonest pattern is an elevation of the IgM with a very low IgE level. When IgE levels are low, skin testing and IgE RAST are of no value. Low IgA predisposes to food allergy, and always suggests the diagnosis. Occasionally, elevations in IgA and IgG are seen in the food allergy complex. High IgG is associated with the more serious immune-mediated diseases, and reflects increased antibody production against unknown antigens. Normal levels of these antibodies do not rule out the diagnosis of food allergy.

12.0.6 Immune Complex Assays

The detection of circulating immune complexes is an important test of the IMED hypothesis. Usually this procedure is reserved for research, and is not routinely employed in patient evaluation. The lab assessment of CIC's tends to be both difficult and expensive. Improvement in techniques and automation is currently making CIC measurement more practical. The most interesting test procedures not only detect CIC's, but also determine which food antigen has complexed with the antibody.[57] A panel of food antigens can now be tested for inclusion in CIC's. This demonstration of food-antigen-containing CIC's gives both the Doctor and patient satisfaction, since the phenomenon of IMED is objectively demonstrated. Unfortunately, we again face the uncertainty principle when we must interpret the test results in terms of dysfunction and disease. We do not yet know how the immune complex correlates with the disease pattern. Immune complexes differ in their size, shape, and biological significance; some may be very dangerous, others benign The dysfunctional results will surely depend on the kind, amount, and frequency of CIC formation. The amount of antigen appearing in the blood, compared with the amount of antibody available, determines the expression of the immunological response. The presence of CIC's tends to increase suppressor effects. The complexities of the immune mesh challenge the thinking of all systems analysts. Food antigens which escape complexing with circulating antibody may be an equal or greater problem than CIC's themselves. Intensive research is needed into these relationships before immune complex assay will be a reliable clinical tool.

12.0.7 Bizarre Food Sensitivity Tests

Muscle testing was one of the first bizarre charades used to demonstrate "food sensitivity". The subject is invited to hold a glass vial containing the test substance and the examiner tests the strength of the other arm which is outstretched. Weakness is interpreted as a food reaction, and the subject is advised to avoid the test substance. Variations on this theme have emerged. A simple resistance meter dressed up in a fancy box (Vega meter) is used to measure skin resistance between a ground plate on which the glass vial is placed, and an "acupuncture point", usually at the thumb web. Increased meter readings are interpreted as a "positive reaction". There is no biology in these maneouvres. A pseudoscience explanatory system referring to "oscillations in the electromagnetic field" confuse the sincere patient with little understanding of physics, electronics, or biology. As one Vega test practitioner promises:

> "This method of diagnosis is based on accurate electrical measurements of the bioelectric potential of the various body systems...The method is quick and effective without the sometimes distressing and lengthy procedures employed in other approaches to this most important aspect of health care."

In another context, these tests would seem a ludicrous charade. What makes the popularity of these shams a serious matter is the suffering of the patients, who are eager for solutions to their chronic problems. A set of dice with food names on their faces would probably be as successful as muscle testing or meter testing in producing good results; any procedure which leads to diet revision with the exclusion of any foods has a chance of success if several common problematic foods are eliminated from the diet.

12.1 Treating Food Allergy

Diet revision therapy (DRT) remains the treatment of choice in all patterns of food allergy. In the immediate hypersensitivity disorders, avoidance of specific foods or food groups removes specific antigens and the problems subside. Most allergists have limited their attention to this pattern, and most published "elimination or allergy" diets are designed only to eliminate specific foods, like milk, or food additives, like sulphites and salicylates. The entire thrust of NP strategy is to resolve the less obvious, more complex disorders by comprehensively reprogramming the diet. Food selection is completely reviewed and revised by beginning again with the safest foods and progressing through the addition of nutritionally desirable and lower risk foods at a slow pace. All symptoms are recorded by the patient and are monitored by a skilled, physician evaluator until a Core Diet of safe foods is established.

Most patients will stabilize with a "Core Diet" consisting of safe foods, defined by eating experiences and monitored with a food-intake-symptom journal. This stability tends to be maintained as long as the restraints of the Core Diet are obeyed. Micronutrients are supplemented, and carbohydrate/fat/protein proportioning is adjusted as needed. A minority of patients display little tolerance to food at all, and often are exquisitely sensitive to airborne chemicals, especially petroleum products, engine exhaust, perfumes, and cigarette smoke. Their symptoms always include brain disturbances, which are often disabling. They seem to have a low dose/frequency threshold for most foods, which limits their food intake to levels below nutritional adequacy. The continued use of an elemental nutrient formula, providing up to 50% of their daily nutrient intake, will often reduce their dysfunction to an acceptable level. Complete vitamin and mineral supplementation is required, although the choice of supplement product is critical, since adverse reactions to casually formulated products are common. Attempts are made to improve tolerance by revision of home and work environments, as well as the use of pharmacological agents directed at modifying GIT function and/or modifying the immune response.

12.1.1 Food Frequency: Sensitization: Rotation

There is a major misunderstanding in popular food allergy books which suggests that new "sensitization" is responsible for symptoms when a food is eaten regularly. This argument is used to support that idea of rotating foods on a 4 5 day schedule. Food immunology tells us another story. Here are the main rules:

1. We are rapidly immunized to any food we eat. We do not have to eat a lot of a food to be "sensitized" to it.

2. The rotation schedule is unlikely to prevent any circulating immune response to incoming antigens, but reduces the total dose of the food ingested over time. This reduced body burden of antigens may the most helpful function of rotation diets.

3. The regular consumption of a "safe" food will not induce new antibody production, but, of course, increases the person's exposure to the IMED possibility of that food.

4. A safe food is presumably safe because it is well-digested and does not contribute an undue body burden of antigenic macromolecules. The rotation of safe food is not necessary.

The dose and frequency of ingesting any food are interdependent variables. The rules for dose/frequency distribution are never easy to establish. In general, higher risk foods (e.g. milk, wheat and other cereal grains, eggs, soy, corn, nuts) are eaten in smaller quantities with a reduced frequency or not at all and lower risk foods (e.g. rice, broccoli, carrots, peas, cauliflower, yams, chicken or turkey) are eaten in increased amounts with increased frequency. For most people, switching to the Core Diets means increasing vegetable intake by 100-300% and significantly reducing intake of North American staple foods - cereal, bread, milk, eggs, beef, corn, potatoes, coffee, tea, alcoholic beverages, and all manufactured, processed foods.

12.1.2 The Yeast Theory

The yeast theory of food allergy has gained unaccountable popularity, and deserves consideration as an ill-conceived theory in the quest to understand food-related illness. The possible role of yeast in causing illness has been popularized by Dr. Crook in the "Yeast Connection"[58] and other books. This theory tries to explain the whole spectrum of food allergy as "yeast allergy". Somehow, the ingestion of diverse food yeasts and unrelated fungi is associated with the overgrowth of candida albicans, a body yeast, which lives in us and on us, as part of our normal collection of microorganisms. The invisible overgrowth of candida in the GIT is supposed to cause all our symptoms. Therapy is designed to kill the yeast with drugs. Avoidance of all fungi in the diet, even mushrooms, which have only the most remote connection with yeasts (both are fungi), is recommended.

Candida yeasts are symbiotic organisms - everyone has lots of them. Yeasts overgrow when conditions are right for them, and cause us distress. You cannot get rid of all of your yeast. You must find an ecological balance, with yeast growing at a controlled rate, below the symptom-producing level. In women, candidal overgrowth is commonly associated with vaginitis. Men may be troubled by yeast overgrowth on their penis or on the skin around the anus and groin. Vaginitis is often provoked or aggrevated by sexual intercourse. Many woman suffer prolonged and mysterious vaginal irritation and pelvic pain. Infection is always assumed, and repeated treatment for candida and other organisms often fails. Seldom is the diagnosis of vaginal allergy considered. The vagina often reacts to circulating food allergens with increased mucus production and secondary candida overgrowth. Milk allergy, for example, commonly triggers vaginitis in both children and adults. High fruit intake is often associated with vaginitis and systemic allergy. Fruit sugars may contribute to candidal overgrowth, but this is not likely in normal women. Diabetic women with elevated body sugar concentrations do suffer candidal overpopulation. Prostaglandins in male semen, and allergic responses to semen and/or sperm may be important contributors to vaginitis. Dr. Wilkins, from Cornell, reported that candida overgrew in the vaginas of women whose immune reponse was supressed by prostaglandin E2.[59] Ibuprofen, a prostaglandin inhibitor, improved the anticandidal response. Prostaglandins were originally discovered in, and named for, secretions of the male prostate gland. Male semen prostaglandins may, in some couples, inhibit the woman's local immune defense. Often, semen proteins or sperm excite female antibody production and set her up for an allergic, inflammatory response. Vaginal candida overgrowth, as everywhere else, is a symptom of another pathological process, and not a cause of it.

Babies often have candidal overgrowth on the diaper area of their skin, producing the most aggressive from of "diaper rash". Oral growth of candida is known as "thrush" and is also common in babies. Infants with inborn errors of amino acid metabolism also display prominent thrush. Candida is very irritating, and is perceived as whitish surface material and marked local inflammation with itching and burning pain. A typical sickly sweet odor is also obvious. Vaginal candida overgrows in response to local changes in microbial flora and immune defense induced by oral contraceptive and antibiotic use. It is common in diabetics with elevated sugar in their secretions, since yeast, like candida, thrive on sugar. Antibiotic use damages the ecology of microorganisms in the bowel and on body surfaces, permitting the overgrowth of candida, and undesirable bacteria. It is reasonable to take oral Nystatin in association with a broad-spectrum antibiotic. Tetracycline, an antibiotic which often promotes candida growth, was once marketed in a capsule which contained Nystatin. Avoidance of antibiotic usage is an even better strategy, especially when antibiotics are often used to treat conditions for which they offer no benefit. Opportunistic growth of candida occurs in people with defective immunity, and can be life-threatening. Metabolites of candida, in increased concentrations, can be toxic, and whole body effects from intestinal overgrowth should be expected. People with demonstrable candida overgrowth should be treated by an attempt to improve the growth of competitive microorganisms, and by the use of the oral antifungal antibiotic, Nystatin. Nystatin should not be used in the absence of direct evidence of candidal overgrowth by lab culture, or in the absence of compelling circumstantial evidence of the problem.

Dr. Crook's program has become rather popular, despite its lack of substance. The desire for a simple, single causes of mysterious illness is understandable in a world of complexity, confusion, and unresolved difficulties. Several points are worth considering:

1. There are many fungi in our food supply. They cause illness by varied and diverse mechanisms. Each fungus should be considered on its own merits and demerits.

2. Immune responses to different fungal antigens tend to different. Cross reactions may exist, but generally these interactions are unkown.

3. The overgrowth of candida should always be interpreted as a symptom of an underlying disorder and not the cause of the disorder.

4. You cannot be tested for candida allergy. Everyone should be sensitive to candidal antigens. The skin test with candida antigen is used as a test of immune-competence. A positive response is usually delayed –the skin reaction is read at 48 hours after injection. If you do not react to candida antigen, something is wrong with your immune response. Immediate reactions (within 30 minutes) to candida antigen injection are difficult to interpret – it does not necessarily mean that "candida allergy" is responsible for your symptoms.

5. The "yeast connection" theory remains ignorant of the diverse mechanisms of adverse reactions to food, and tends interfere with the proper understanding of these mechanisms; it is, therefore, counter–productive. The symptoms attributed to candida are typical of the wide spectrum of adverse reactions to food, and should not be interpreted as having a single cause.

6. People who accept the "yeast connection" are encouraged by product advertisements to buy easy solutions to chronic health problems, which really require responsible, dedicated, and persistent efforts to resolve. They are encouraged to use drugs, like the antibiotics Nystatin and Nizoral, without appreciating the risk of side effects and toxicity. Both antibiotics are potentially toxic. Nystatin is relatively safe only if it is not absorbed from the intestine. The risk of significant absorption increases as the dose of Nystatin is increased and prolonged. Nizoral is routinely absorbed, and has been implicated in hepatitis deaths. The recommended use of Nizoral is limited by this potential toxicity to serious fungal infections not resolved by other means. Other products are now sold and advertised nationally as candida cures. All of these products, including acidophillus, garlic, caprylic acid, herbs, animal gland derivatives, and vitamins, are not likely to influence candidal growth and do not contribute to the proper treatment of food allergy.

Chapter 13

COMPULSIVE EATING & ADDICTIVE BEHAVIOR

Our story of food-behavior interactions becomes even more complex when we observe the many problems children and their families experience when they attempt diet revision. This chapter is an introduction to the puzzling phenomena of disordered eating patterns, withdrawal effects, compliance difficulties, compulsive eating, "cheating", and giving up.

Often children with food allergy or other food-related illness are abnormal eaters. They are described as "picky" or "fussy" in their food selection. They may refuse to eat many foods, specializing in 6-10 favorites, or they may eat continuously and compulsively, growing fat. Often children go through food fads, eating one or two foods almost monotonously for weeks or months, then switching to another selection. Children with more serious forms of food allergy tend to be "food specialists", often undereating and tending to be below average in height and weight. Fat children also have food allergy and may also be food specialists, but overeat continously or binge episodically on staple foods - milk, cheese, bread, crackers, meat, potatoes, fruit - as well as sweets and ice cream.

Most parents report "sugar" cravings and/or binging. "Sugar" means a wide range of candies, cookies, desserts, baked goods, pop, ice cream, and junk food. The sugar is only one component among many that may cause trouble. But these foods definitely trigger strong cravings and compulsive or binge eating. Cravings for milk, bread, cheese, peanuts, fruit, or potato chips are as common as cravings for sweets. Even children with obvious milk allergy, with a protective aversion to drinking milk, will compulsively eat cheese or ice cream, maintaining their milk-allergic illness.

We recognize an underlying "addictive" cycle to the abnormal eating behaviors observed in children. The exact cause of the addictive cycle is not known, but is clearly not just sugar or any other single food ingredient.

Thousands of other molecular species in the food supply are also implicated, including "Agent X", an unknown environmental contaminant. We are certain, however, that certain substances in the children's food supply, act like addictive drugs and trigger cycles of food cravings and compulsive eating. A compulsion is an irresistable behavior, an action that defies conscious control. The worst afflicted children will not follow the core diet (or any other food control) voluntarily. They are driven by uncontrollable urge to get and eat forbidden foods. They must be managed carefully, with compassion, weaned from addictive foods and then maintained in control by abstaining from addictive foods. They are similar in every respect to an alcoholic or drug addict. If their compulsive eating is not corrected it is possible that they will tend toward a life of addictive behavior, in the worst case, becoming alcoholics and/or drug abusers.

The success of the Core Diet depends on guiding children through a initial withdrawal period of 5-10 days. During withdrawal, access to old familiar foods is withdrawn and the Phase 1 Core Diet foods are offered. Food cravings and compulsive food-seeking behavior is to be expected. Frustration occurs whenever one of our drives is blocked. The craving child is frustrated when a craved food is denied. Many of the children I work with follow the Core Diet with little difficulty and get better uneventfully. They respond well to the explanation and reassurance of their parents. Evidence of withdrawal symptoms and frustration disappears by day 5-10. For many children, this "clearing" effect is the beginning of a whole new mode of functioning. Clearing tends to open children's appetite to new foods, and, with a little reward and encouragement, Core Diet foods start looking attractive.

Other children have more difficulty and continue to eat reactive foods (with or without their parents' knowledge) and follow a roller coaster path of physical and mental disturbance. The children who tend to stay in trouble have an antisocial, addictive behavioral profile with sugar cravings, compulsive eating, and limit their food intake to a few favorite foods and beverages - usually high in milk, wheat, and egg proteins along with sugar. They go through obvious withdrawal in the first week on the Core Diet, often with angry, tearful protests, and refuse to eat Core Diet foods. The worst of them will go to any length to maintain their old food habits - lying, cheating, and stealing fordidden foods are not out of the question. These children also tend to radical mood shifts, displays of anger, and often alienate their family, school and friends by angry, aggressive behavior. Often one parent - usually the parent who does not actively seek a solution for the child's problem - displays a similar pattern and may contribute to "cheating". An aggressive child will promote conflict between parents who are not in complete agreement about food selection and management. The compulsive parent will "give-in" to the child's demands or will, in the worst case, seek the child's favor by offering forbidden foods. It is easy to buy a child's favor with pop, ice cream, and chocolate bars. It is difficult to seek the child's health and happiness by opposing impulsive, pleasure-seeking, and offering instead safe Core Diet foods.

Complete abstinence from foods that trigger compulsive eating is the only way to avoid recurrence of the addictive cycle. If you reduce the opportunity to eat wrong foods at home or cheat away from home, you encourage your child to follow the Core Diet food list, without exceptions, and the cravings go away. If food exceptions are made, even every 3 or 4 days, the incoming problem may be sufficient to sustain cravings, and spoil the clearing effect. If one or both parents continue to have problems managing their own food cravings and compulsions, the attempt at diet revision usually fails.

13.0.1 A Letter from a Child in Withdrawal

I received the following letter from a nine year patient after he had been on the Core Diet for a few days. He is in withdrawal. His remarks are poignant and somehow epitomize the predicament of both children and adults as they face changes in habitual patterns:

"Dear Dr. Gislason,

This program is driving me nuts. Yesterday I went to a Birthday and I couldn't have any of the food. I moped. and in 17 days It's my birthday. And what is a birthday if the birthday boy can't have his cake?

I want real food, pizza, hot dogs, hamburger, lasagna, corn, meatballs, ribbs. I understand its for my health but at times I almost eat bread and things. But I know if I eat bread and I am so close to a week that I can eat something else that I'll spoil it. and I don't want to do that. do I have to put up with this for life? I'm sick of the stuff I get.

Sincearly yours,

Gerald"

I think Gerald should get a Smithsonian award for his efforts. His suffering is genuine as he experiences withdrawal and his mini-grieving process begins for the loss of favorite foods. I know that he is enduring withdrawal from the foods he misses. We can empathize with his feelings, and encourage him to push through this temporary distress toward a new state of well-being. A successful child quickly passes through this phase and starts eating Core Diet foods, often with increased appetite.

13.1 The Addictive Loop

One of the great puzzles of the food allergy business is the curious and biologically perverse phenomenon of craving and compulsive eating of injurious foods and drinks. Cravings may be interpreted as urges to find missing nutrients, but the foods found in compulsive food-searches are not biologically correct. Instead, food cravings are a symptom of an addictive loop, linking appetite to foods which contain addictive substances, chemical stressors, or allergenic triggers. The term "addictive food allergy" has become popular. The puzzle of cravings and compulsions is solvable by good biological thinking. We can look for molecular information contained in food which programs recursive loops (RCL) and keeps people locked into self-destructive cycles.

Bulimia is a rapidly emerging illness complex of food cravings, compulsive eating, food binges, with attempts to fast, purge, or vomit. Bulimia is reported in increasing numbers of adolescents and young adults, more often female than male, with alarming implications. Psychological explanations of this growing aberration are easily conconcted out of psychosomatic myths and idle opinion. Are the pyschological explanations valid in any way? Or are there biological forces in our environment and food supply that disorder brain control of appetite and eating behaviors? Compulsive eating occurs when the brain's appetite system malfunctions. Self-induced vomiting or laxative administration are deliberate acts to minimize the consequences of compusive eating. Something in the food supply causes the disorganized eating pattern, and other behavior problems follow in a complex manner.

A variety of interesting explanations for compulsive or "binge" eating may be proposed. The basic behavior may be described as a recursive loop - eating substance X triggers increased appetite for more substance X. Everyone has experienced some degree of "binge" eating. Peanuts or any of the ubiquitous snack foods are likely to catch most people in a hand-to-mouth loop. Alcoholic beverages catch too many people in a viscious, self-destructive cycle. Chocolate confections and sugar containing-foods trap others. Once trained to binge on a food, the sight or smell of the "fix" will trigger a craving for it. Tasting the first mouthful of a binge food often triggers uncontrolled binging. Food cravings follow body rhythms, and may change seasonally.

The possibility that food contains specific molecular species that induce true addiction is supported by clinical observations and neurochemical research. Since adverse reactions to food are related to compulsive eating of the same food, the possibilty of addiction to the reactive process must be considered. Drug-like, addictive molecules are "Recursive-Loop-Inducers" (RCLI). These substances act on brain cells, establishing new set-points which then demand their continuing presence.

Closed-looping locks us into recursive, repeating behaviors, cravings, and compulsions, usually with negative brain consequences, disorder, and ill-health. Human behavior is determined to an alarming degree by addictive-molecules. Elaborate habit-structures are built around the single goal of delivering a regular supply of addictive molecules. The drives to maintain brain concentrations of addictive substances are organized in the older core brain or limbic structures which do not ask consciousness for permission to operate. The core brain is characterized by a low level consciousness, and a high level of automaticity. The experience of cravings for, and drives to find addictive molecules is, therefore, profoundly disturbing to us.

Most insightful people will describe a "split" in their personality; automatic seeking behaviors take over, and consciousness simply monitors the behavioral events which follow. The idea of "willpower" is difficult to substantiate, since there does not seem to be a brain procedure which reaches from high-level thinking down into the machine level programming, where automatic behaviors are produced. Parents report rapid dramatic mood shifts in their children and describe angry, defiant behavior. We associate the negative behavior with specific foods that are craved and eaten compulsively. When a child clears on the Core Diet all evidence of the negative personality may disappear until a reactive food is eaten again.

The characteristic of addictive behavior is the stereotypic search for the food, beverage, or drug which supplies a specific addictive molecule or a substitute. This Search Mode (SM) may be concealed by layers of social behavior that are more or less acceptible in adults who are generally free to select the foods and beverages. Children generally have more supervision and often must break family rules to indulge their cravings. When we impose the Core Diet rules, the constraints may to too strict for an addictive child and the rules may be broken by concealing the evidence. A strict parent tends to produce more cheating behavior with lying and stealing to cover up the compulsive food-seeking. A non confrontational approach is best. There is no punishment for "cheating" and always rewards for following the proper Core Diet plan.

Successful programs for reducing addictive behavior work on external behavioral structures first to withdraw from the addictive substances, and then to maintain succesful abstinence. The control of addiction is strategic, rather than moral. Whenever possible remove temptation. Family cooperation is essential. Offer alternatives to reactive or trigger foods. A chocolate chip cookie may be dynamite, but a rice-flour cookie with carob may be OK.

13.1.1 Withdrawal

The association between addiction and illness is close and puzzling. A neurochemical thesis suggests that addictive molecules work directly or indirectly through interaction with brain systems responsible for regulating our body processes, our appetites, and our consciousness. The craving triggers are addictive substances in food that alter the activity of neurons so that their presence is then required to maintain homeostasis. Further craving triggers input is achieved through the appetitive system which drives behavior toward the goal of getting some more (cravings and compulsions).

Learning occurs on a molecular level in the brain. The craving triggers act as positive reinforcers of specific food choices, and neurons adapt to their presence. When a neural system learns to function in the presence of craving triggers, tolerance is established, and the business of living goes on, as long as the food containing the trigger substances is eaten regularly. Often children experience withdrawal symptoms within 3-4 hours of not eating their addictive food. They become restless and irritable, and may go to considerable trouble to get their fix if it is not immediately available. If the craving triggers's are suddenly withdrawn, the neural system malfunctions, over-reacts, oscillates, and produces a major withdrawal disturbance. These mini-withdrawal episodes are often blamed on "hypoglycemia". Seldom is low blood sugar involved. The disturbance is much more profound and occurs within the complex computations of the brain.

With continued abstinence from the trigger food, the neural over-reaction settles down to a more stable level of function. With complete abstinence from problem foods, 5-10 days is required for the brain-emitted disturbance to settle.

Slow withdrawal of offending foods reduces the severity of withdrawal. However, slow withdrawal is more difficult because the craving triggers food maintains cravings and compulsions which preclude control of food selection. All addictive cycles present you with the same conundrum: allow your child to suffer "cold-turkey" withdrawal and get out of the recursive loop quickly; or suffer less acute withdrawal and experience prolonged cravings and compulsive eating behaviors. Continuing stability of new food habits requires complete abstinence from the foods containing the addicting craving triggers's. Food addiction is surprisingly similar to narcotic or alcohol addiction.

We can predict that food addiction programs, well-learned on the molecular level after a few repetitions, are linked by classical and operant conditioning to sights, smells, sounds, faces, and so on. This conditioned linking mechanisms allows circumstances and events to take over as triggers for compulsive eating behaviors. Often the first smell or taste of foods containing craving triggers's triggers an eating binge that exceeds voluntary control. This context-dependent addictive behavior must be recognized before behavioral modification succeeds in correcting compulsive eating disorders. The concept of craving triggers's can be elaborated in many directions. An aromatic (strong smell and taste) molecule which is linked by operant conditioning to a compulsive behavior becomes an addictive trigger (craving triggers) by association, and not by its own chemical action.

13.1.2 Narcotics in Digests of Food Proteins

Several researchers have pursued a very important discovery: that the digestion of food proteins from milk and wheat produces substances having narcotic drug-like activity. These substances have been termed "exorphins".[60] Digests of milk proteins also are opioid peptides.[61] The human brain effects of exorphins have not yet been studied, but are likely to contribute to the mental disturbances and appetite disorders which routinely accompany food-related illness. The possibility that exorphins are addictive in some people is a fascinating lead which needs further exploration.

Another mechanism, similar to dependency on food-derived neuroactive peptides like the exorphins, would be a dependency on gastrointestinal peptides, released from the GIT during digestion. Deficiencies in the GIT production of regulatory addictive peptides, such as endorphins, would likely be associated with cravings and compulsions to increase food ingestion. There are a large number of gut-regulatory peptides feeding back to brain control centers to form the brain-gut axis. The information flow between the gut and brain is likely critical in regulating feeding behaviors.

13.1.3 Sugar

The most common food sugar is sucrose, an A-2 molecule, which digests to glucose and fructose, normal A-1 molecules. The presence of sugar in food increases the desirability of the food, and increases the incidence of addictive behavior. Food manufacturers realize that sugar is good for repeat business and regularly add sugar to all their food products. The addictive action of sugars must be biochemically mediated, probably by the influence of glucose on appetite-computing neurons. Glucose is a positive molecular reinforcer of feeding behaviors which bring it into the hypothalamic nuclei of the brain. Glucose may indirectly determine neurotransmitter synthesis by regulating the competition among amino acids for entry into the brain. The sugar load in a meal also influences the digestive sensors, which release GIT regulators, and feedback to the brain as second level positive reinforcers of the feeding behavior. Behaviorists would argue that the taste of sugar is positive reinforcement at the behavioral level for the selection and consumption of high-sugar food. They would point out all the behavioral conditioning, linking high-sugar foods to pleasure and reward. A more general theory would include a variety of mechanisms underlying compulsive sugar-food ingestion. Learned behavior, pleasure-seeking, and molecular conditioning would all merge toward the cravings and compulsions which sugar promotes.

Diet revision always must include sugar constraint, if only to reduce cravings and compulsive behavior which interfere with conscious intentions to regulate food choices. I am convinced that sugar is not the cause of hyperactivity. Sugar seems to increase the effects of the other food problems that do cause hyperactivity, however. I suggest to parents that if sugar is used in moderation with perfectly safe foods, expect no important difficulities. It is not necessary, nor desirable to use sugar substitutes.

13.1.4 Addiction to the Reactive Mechanism

The links between the mechanisms of food allergy and addiction need better biological explanation. Patients with adverse reactions to foods (ARF), allergic and otherwise, regularly crave the foods that hurt them! We might ask: do adverse food reactions release addictive molecules or otherwise condition us to repeat the ingesting behavior which triggers the food reaction? Circulating mediators released in the process of an allergic reaction are many and complex in their body actions. There are many different peptides, prostaglandins, and neurotransmitters, such as norepinephrine, serotonin, and acetylcholine. It is possible that a food reaction releases mediators which act as positive reinforcement of the food-seeking brain mechanism, even though the net effect of eating the food is injurious. If you are conditioned to seek the allergic reaction because of addiction to mediators, we can say that you become addicted to the process of illness itself!

The habituating effects of addictive molecules in the food may only be coincidentally linked to the disease mechanism. For example, someone might crave ice cream as a reward food because it tastes good and because eating ice cream is linked with many positive connotations from childhood onward. But, what if the milk content of the ice cream causes a delayed allergic response? The connection between the food and the symptoms is ignored for a long time because the immediate reward of eating the delicious ice cream reinforces our craving (desire to do it again), and the negative effects of the adverse reaction is too delayed to be linked to the ice cream. The automatic conditioning link which should unconsciously register an aversion to injurious food does not operate unless the reactive effects occur within a short time of the eating experience. The conscious recognition that the food can produce the symptoms experienced requires sustained intellectual effort and significant learning. The association between the pleasureable mouth experiences and the later body disturbances allows illness-causing food habits to go undetected, and to persevere for years.

13.1.5 Addiction and Tolerance

Tolerance to the effects of any substance is a feature of addiction to it. Tolerance represents a volume control on a reactive body system which gets turned down or off. The volume adjustment is achieved by an active brain process. Another possible explanation of the food reaction-craving link lies with the phenomenon of tolerance to stressors. The ability to learn both allergic reactions and compensatory defense regulation has been demonstrated in experimental animals, and is evident in my patient studies.

Brain regulation of body states is not passive. The human brain is not a system which simply waits for something to happen and then reacts. Instead, the brain functions in expectancy-modes (EXM), learning to anticipate regularly occuring events. Expectancy-modes have also been called "feedforward" mechanisms. If we regularly eat a food containing molecular stressors, an EXM event is learned. A defence adjustment is emitted by our brain in clock-like anticipation of the recurrent food challenge. If the challenge event does not occur, the anticipatory EXM is experienced as a disturbance. This disturbance is equivalent to withdrawal from RCL's. Behaviors are then established to avoid the experience of disappointed EXM states. The effect is pseudo-addiction. Or, in other words, we learn to stabilize at an unhealthy point of chronic reactivity, emitting defense behaviors as we go.

The state of many "normal" children and adults could be described as "dysfunctional, but adapted" - a relatively stable, defensive state, holding toxins, allergens, and event-stressors in check. Unfortunately, our efforts to make things better by diet revision or any other major shift in habit-patterns disturb the stable adaptation. In other words, the quest for a new healthier adaptation sends us on a wobbly course for at least a few days, and sometimes a few weeks. I often tell parents and children to imagine they are in a prison (adaptive dysfunctional state) and to get out you have to make a run for it. Thoughtful parents appreciate the difficulties of making a run for it, and offer sympathy and support without any punishment, admonishment, or dire predictions of life-long deprivation.

Chapter 14

FOOD, LEARNING, BEHAVIOR

Children grow and change continuously. Every day they face new and challenging experiences. Their bodies and brains mature progressively, permitting an ever-widening scope of learning, emotional responses, physical coordination and skill. Since they are new to the world and learning continuously, they are always exceeding their competence and skill and need our support and help.

Our genetic program contains a structural blueprint that determines our look, size, and basic personality. The genetic program also contains a developmental sequence. Not all developmental sequences are the same; children show great variation in their ability to learn at different stages. Some children are physically adept, others are clumsy and awkward. Girls tend to do better in language skills during the first decade than boys. Boys prefer rough and tumble play and tend to fight. There is a subgroup of children, more boys than girls, who have special difficulty with language skills and tend to be physically hyperactive. They are restless and dysfunctional in regimented classrooms, but may do well if allowed to be very physically active, to be exploratory, and to concentrate on constructional skills. Often behavioral abnormalities and learning difficulties reflect a mismatch between adult expectations and the readiness of the child's brain to learn. All children thrive on success, as measured by adult and peer group approval. If a child is given a task which he or she is not yet ready to perform, failure leaves a lasting imprint of doubt and low self-esteem. Much childhood suffering could be alleviated by more biologically appropriate task assignment at school and at home. A regimented classroom may not be a suitable environment for children with learning difficulties. Often learning ability improves after physical training of balance and coordination through sports, music, dance, and specific "sensory integration" exercises.

14.0.1 Old Genetic Program Meets New Foods

A child's food supply may influence learning, social adaptation, and personality developments. Social maladaptations, including juvenile deliquency, drug abuse, unemployment, and psychiatric illness can be caused by problems in the food supply.

Ronald Bobner and associates reviewed nutritional disorders, linked to behavioral and learning problems in children.[62] In their introduction they state:

> "Millions of dollars are spent annually on special education programs for children whose severe behavior disorders prevent them from participating in the regular school setting despite average or above average intellectual capacity. a growing body of research indicates that some of these behavioral disorders are related to nutritional problems."

Many factors are considered in the literature including nutrient deficiencies, toxic heavy metals and food allergy. We recognize a strong correlation between patterns of physical ilness and learning-behavioral problems, which suggest that food allergies are important contributors to the most serious problems. We are particulary concerned with increasing numbers of children who are especially aggressive with antisocial behavior, and serious mood swings. Sick children who behave badly create a ripple effect of disturbances in their families, neighborhoods and classrooms. We assume there are a complex, interacting set of possible problems with food-body-brain interactions. The following list summarizes the more obvious causes of brain dysfunction in children.

Negative Brain Effects of Food Choices
1. Nutrient Deficiencies
2. Nutrient Excesses
3. Nutrient Disproportion
4. Toxic Effects
    - Intrinsic Substances
    - Additives
    - Chemical Contaminants
5. Metabolic Abnormalities
6. Food Allergy
7. Proteins and Peptides
8. Drug Effects
    - Intrinsic Psychoactive Susbtances
    - Additives
9. Colon Flora Metabolites and Toxins

Since almost every atom in the child's body entered via the mouth, normal development requires a tight match between the child's genetic program and food supply. It makes perfect biological sense to look at the food supply when children are not growing, developing, and behaving normally.

14.0.2 Somatopsychic Medicine

Pyschosomatic theories, in my opinion, are basically wrong. What is really going on is the other way around. Body-brain events produce mental events - real, practical things, especially material, entering body-brain through the mouth are very important in determining mental events. This is "Somatopsychics". Our mental and emotional status is strongly determined by food and beverages.

The role of foods in creating sick, disturbed children has been seriously underestimated. The role of a variety of food allergic mechanisms in causing common, specific, patterns of learning and behavioral dysfunction is generally not known or is even denied. One of my clinical psychologist colleagues, Chuck Bates, wrote frankly about his experiences in an instruction manual he provided to his clients. His remarks are worth considering.[63]

> "My own case history exemplifi es many of the fundamental principles (of Diet Revision Therapy), and since this technology did more for my mental health than all of the clinical psychology I have learned, put together, my story is a good starting point. As a boy I was diagnosed as having spring pollen and house dust allergie s. I sniffled and sneezed continuously, and years of desensitizing injections didn't seem to help. I continued to have attacks into adulthood. I was a moody and irritable teenager, experiencing great difficulty concentrating on my studies. My

marks disappointed those aware of my high I.Q. In my late teens I experienced severe clinical depression. As an adult, my depression moderated considerably, but took other forms...frequent fatigue attacks... muddied, clouded consciousness a good percent of the time I sat there in a daze, barely able to participate in conversations... I had frequent food cravings and was always at least 20 pounds overweight despite constant dieting. I went on pizza binges, washed down with quarts of milk. Every morning I coughed up mucus. I had insomnia and nightmares. I usually felt jumpy and impatient. I experienced constant flatulence, heartburn, gas pains, indigestion, and diarrhea. I attributed my moodiness to being a spoiled child, and beyond that I had no awareness that anything else was amiss.

"Using (Diet Revision Therapy) technology a new me emerged. All of my symptoms disappeared. I experienced a previously unknown mental clarity and ability to concentrate. My moods, especially my irritability disappeared."

Food, as body input, is understood as the substrate of body-mind, the foundation level, which permits or denies healthy function at higher levels of integration. Immune interaction with food components offer an enormously complex set of abnormal possibilities. Food allergy is therefore one of the most important models of pathological food-brain interactions. Dr. Aas, a Norwegian allergist and researcher, remarked at the Marabou symposium on "Food Sensitivity"[64] :

"In my institute I am the only experimental monkey that we have and from several passive transfer experiments on myself, with occasional rather severe reactions, I am the first to admit that allergic reactions are accompanied with intellectual and emotional disturbances. If you have not experienced that, I ask you to be a volunteer in my laboratory."

14.0.3 Disturbed Behavior

Food allergy is diagnosed in infants by recognizing the typical signs and symptoms discussed throughout the book. In this chapter, the connection between physical problems and mental-emotional problems will be emphasized.

In infants and children, disturbed behavior is a sensitive indicator of food allergy and other forms of food related illness Physical symptoms and disturbed behavior go together. The mother of a food allergic infant has a frustrating and difficult task of caring for an irritable, often screaming, and sleepless infant with itching-erupted skin, vomiting, bowel cramps, diarrhea, and other discomforts which they are unable to express except by crying, squirming, screaming, often throughout the night. Mother often feels guilty about her non-maternal tired, confused, angry reactions to her agitated, disturbed infant. Her guilt is particularly severe if she does not understand the origin of the infant's problem and receives inappropriate advice from professionals, family, or friends. Rapid, decisive changes in the infant's food supply usually resolve the problems within a few days! *Behavior disturbance in infancy promises more problems to come unless the corrections are made in the child's food supply!*

As children develop hyperactive behavior often emerges and is linked to temper tantrums, moodiness, crying, fighting, defiance, and low self esteem. Sometimes the hyperactive behavior is outrageous. Parents describe the worst behaviors with colorful phrases - "bouncing off the walls", "demolition derby","leaping from the chandeliers", " absolutely out of control... insane". Bizarre, repeating, obsessional behaviors are often reported - rocking, head banging, pacing, repeating spoken phrases, grunting, snorting, and rituals with toys, dolls and pets. We occasionally see children who are described as "retarded" or "autistic". Many of the hyperactive children cannot get along with their friends and siblings - they tend to be impulsive, demanding, argumentative, and easily frustrated - their anger may be expressed physically with shouting, punching, kicking and biting.

The same children often have difficulty in school, failing to learn, disrupting classrooms, and failing to sustain healthy friendships. If their behavior is not corrected by proper diet revision they develop antisocial attitudes and habits. The worst afflicted, after years of family and school conflict, develop sociopathic personalities - social outcasts, glib liars with little or no affection or feeling for other people- restless, impulsive, adolescents, often addicted to food, alcohol, and drugs.

The trials and tribulations of parents are many, and often parents feel guilty and confused about their children's antics when expertise in behavioral management would make no difference at all. These children often have body input problems or food allergy. Food allergic illness is associated with behavioral disturbances which grow by a natural evolution of dysfunction and social maladaptation into major life problems. To understand this better, we need a sophisticated whole-system's view of childrens' problems. Their problems are biological, not "psychological".

Mind and body are one interacting whole. The most likely direction of problem flow is from cellular-biochemical disturbance to mental disturbance, rather than from mental disturbance to cellular-biochemical dysfunction. Without healthy body input attempts to improve mental and emotional status of children by social and behavioral means ultimately fail.

14.1 Neurobiology of Psychic Energy

Psychic energy (PsyE) is the stuff of consciousness, arousal, attention, emotion and human action. Psychic energy is the force that wakes us up, connects us to the world with desires and drives, and brings us into action. In our practical biological model, PsyE is first understood as function level of brain activity. Disorders of psychic energy and arousal may be described as attention deficits, hyperactivity, unstable moods, temper tantrums, and depression. A brief excerpt from a more complete essay on this subject is included to give you basic understanding of these problems in biological terms.

14.1.1 Origin of Psychic Energy

The brain is an electrochemical information processing system, requiring a well-regulated, continuous supply of oxygen and nutrients to function properly. Unlike other organs, the brain does not store oxygen and nutrients, and is therefore critically dependent on the molecular flow brought to it by its blood supply. Brain activity makes high energy demands on body metabolism. At rest, the brain consumes at least 50% of its peak operating energy consumption, manifesting a continuous readiness to act. In contrast, resting skeletal muscle consumes less that 10% of peak energy consumption. Even in sleep, vigorous brain activity during the dream (rapid-eye-movement) sleep consumes peak energy. The influence of the day's body input on sleep is clinically observable, and the quality of sleep is critical in establishing proper energy and function for the next day. Poor sleep means poor PsyE and contributes to on-going fatigue, mental and emotional aberrations during the day.

14.1.2 Moods as Arousal Modulation

The arousal activity of the core brain brings us to consciousness and directs our activities. A set of carrier frequencies provides basic arousal and is modulated by other monitoring activities in the core brain. We tend to feel this modulation as "mood". Mood is elusive. There are no specific contents of mood, since it is simply a modulation of PsyE. The brain procedures which select mood, however, also seem to select cognitive programs, appropriate to that mood. Thus, thinking will shift, often dramatically and inexplicably, from positive to negative thought structures as the mood vectors shift.

Color metaphors are often used to describe mood; black seems naturally suited to the negative moods, associated with night, anxiety, fear, and death. Happy moods are not white, but light colors; the purest sky blue is chosen in oriental symbolism to represent the clear untroubled mind. The sense of not-being-well is "dysphoria". The sense of all-being-well is "euphoria". If a high energy state is modulated by dysphoric signals, suffering is the result - dread, despair, doom. If the same high energy state is modulated by euphoric signals, the "high" experience of bliss, oneness, ecstasy is the reward. As with all our brain functions, these signals can intermodulate in a jumble of confused moods; agitated depression may occur, or a hyperactive, manic state with high energy, overly-optimistic interpretations, but with dysphoric feelings, spoiling the manic high.

14.1.3 Moods and Thinking

The cognitive styles and structures attached to different moods may so distinct and dissociated from other cognitive structures that different personalities seem to emerge in the same person. The splitting of the personality is often reported by my insightful adult patients, most of whom would otherwise be thought of as ordinary, sane people. Many parents describe a "Jekyll and Hyde" transformation of their children. The flip-flop, abrupt style of mood transition is typical of food reactions. The surprising fact is that different foods have such a profound impact on mood, and therefore, on the cognitive styles of individuals. Mood determination is closely linked to brain procedures which regulate all body functions, and it does make biological sense to observe close relationships between food, mood-arousal disorders, digestive and immune dysfunctions.

A continuous flow of proper nutrients is essential to good PsyE. Just as important is the absence of interference with proper brain function by avoidance of the inappropriate input of problematic molecular species. When PsyE is decreased and mood vectors shift to the dysphoric, we diagnose "Depression". As depression worsens, emotions blacken, tears flow, anger increases, pleasure and interest vanish. Thinking is usually disturbed, with reduced attention span, distractability, and increased difficulty in remembering recent events. The experience is the result of brain dysfunction, biochemically induced.

Children display paradoxical states, combining depression with irritability or hyperactivity. They may be hyperactive, loud, and aggressive while failing to pay attention, learn, relate to others, or feel pleasure. This paradoxical arousal state is unstable and often explodes in a temper tantrum, or other irrational, inappropriate behaviors.

14.1.4 Brain Chemistry

Most discussions of mood or arousal disorders in the neurochemical literature talk about neurotransmitters in tidy little boxes, hidden away in the brain. The assumption is that brain chemistry has its own internal rules and is not influenced by things coming into the system from the outside. Food is inconveniently complex, and is therefore almost never discussed in the neuropsychiatric literature. When mental disorders are attributed to "chemical imbalances in the brain", we are not supposed to think of food coming into the system, but of some mysterious internal problem that operates for its own reasons.

The alternative way of thinking (the correct way) is that "chemical imbalances in the brain" are caused by the wrong body input, and can be corrected by appropriate diet revision.

Neurobiological models of depression are based on observations of altered neurotransmitter synthesis and function in the brains of laboratory animals. The action of antidepressant drugs in these animal models has provided important leads toward the understanding of the different brain systems involved in producing and regulating PsyE.

14.1.5 SANDOH, the Arousal System

Consciousness depends on spontaneously emitted pulses from brain stem neurons which ascend in a complex mesh of activating circuits to awaken neurons in the limbic system and cerebral cortex. Without this ascending activation, we lapse into a coma. Sleep is an organized inhibition of the ascending activation, orchestrated by neurons within the activation complex. Honest fatigue is a normal prelude to sleep, and represents the increasing activity of sleep-inducing neurons. Some of the sleep-inducing neurons use serotonin as the transmitter and malfunction when its precursor, tryptophan, is deficient; thus bedtime doses of this amino acid promote sleep. Extra tryptophan during the day may make you feel tired and dopey. Children with food allergy often have disturbed sleep.

We can imagine the arousal system in our core brain as a meshwork of six interacting tree-like systems. There are at least six different neurotransmitters operating this system and dozens of modulating substances, especially hormones and immune system mediators. Three of the systems are the core of the activation system, and are identified with the neurotransmitters Serotonin, Acetylcholine, and Norepinephrine (SAN). The accessory activation system utilizes Dopamine, Opiates, and Histamine (DOH). The combined frequency-modulated synthesizer, SANDOH, acts to determine our consciousness, reactivity, attention, vigilance, and emotional experience.

14.1.6 The Role of Amino Acids

Norepinephrine and dopamine are made from the amino acids phenylalanine, tyrosine, and L-dopa. L-dopa is used to treat patients with parkinson's disease who often experience extreme fatigue, depression, and slowing of all movement. These amino acids taken orally in pill form are not powerful antidepressants, but may have a contributing role in a well thought-out neurochemical recipe. Rather simple-minded theories have linked the ingestion of foods containing more or less of the amino acids tryptophan, phenylalanine and tyrosine with mood changes. According to Judith Wurtman changes in arousal can be explained by carbohydrate/protein ratios using the simple idea that high protein foods are stimulating and "carbohydrate" foods are sedative becase they increase the synthesis of serotonin from tryptophan. In Wurtman's book "Managing Your Mind Through Food"[65] we are encouraged to eat high protein foods "...when your brain's supply of dopamine and norepinephrine is beginning to run short..." Suggested meals include whole-grain bread, skim milk, cottage cheese, and eggs.

Our clinical experience would suggest just the opposite. The high protein foods are potentially allergenic and may effect brain function through complicated immune-mediated mechanisms - not simply their content of amino acids! Many allergic children would be sedated, or disabled with poor concentration and decreased memory if they attempted to eat wheat, eggs and/or milk. Some children would be paradoxically hyperactive.

These three common foods have proven to be the most important contributors to childrens' food allergy problems, learning, and behavioral difficulties.

Theories which stress the activity of single nutrients within the complex mix of various foods are always wrong. Living systems are always more complex than anyone can imagine.

14.1.7 AcetylCholine

Our principle arousal network uses acetylcholine (Ach) as the transmitter. Increasing Ach activity arouses our thinking, memory, and computational abilities, but too much may make us feel depressed. Most antidepressant drugs block acetylcholine circuits, and, if taken in overdose, produce stupor and coma by Ach blockade. In this drug-overdose mode, the same Ach drug, physostigmine, awakens the comatose patient immediately, although the effect is short-lived and must be repeated. The administration of choline, the Ach precursor, to improve memory may also produce fatigue or depression. Common insecticides (Malathion, Parathion, EPN, Schradan), which contaminate our food supply and poison farm-workers, are related to "nerve gases" (Saran, Soman), which all act on the Ach system. They block the breakdown of Ach, so that it accumulates and prevents further Ach messages to get through. The result is respiratory failure and convulsions, quickly fatal if the dose is high enough. The role of pesticide residues in our food supply in causing mental and emotion symptoms is unknown, but anyone who doubts a possible connection should review their neurochemistry.

14.1.8 Norepinephrine

Norepinephrine (NE) is another arousal transmitter, found in the locus coeruleus and its ascending circuits within the arousal complex. In rats, the legitimate stress of painful, uncontrollable electrical shocks induces depression promptly, and is associated with early depletion of NE in the locus coeruleus.[66] An underproduction of NE, because of enzyme deficiency, or lack of nutrient substrates, may lead to depression. Some antidepressants, especially imipramine, selectively alter the synthesis of NE, but paradoxical experimental results tell us that the therapeutic changes are not simply increasing one transmitter, but rather influencing the net arousal balance in the mesh. Imipramine is the grandmother of the family of "tricyclic" antidepressants. Imipramine has at least a triple action on NE,

Ach, and Histamine circuits. Despite its prominent anti-Ach side effects, it is a very useful drug, which has rescued many of my patients from dysfunction and despair. Children with bed wetting are often safely treated with imipramine. Children with depression and attention-deficit disorder with hyperactivity also often respond favorably to imipramine at doses of 10-50 mg at bedtime. Careful application of the Core Diet usually replaces all drug therapy, however, and is by far the better mode of therapy.

14.1.9 Stimulants

Stimulants, including caffeine, cocaine, ritalin, and amphetamines, act in a NE-increasing mode, with temporary activation of PsyE, and sense of well-being. They also influence the dopamine system. The repeated use of these drugs leaves the overstimulated circuits in a state of confusion, with aberrancies in PYSE supply, and disturbed thinking, feeling, and behavior. Withdrawal from these drugs is associated with other marked disturbances that may take weeks to settle.

Newton's second law adapts perfectly to our brain: for every neurochemical force applied, there is an equal and opposite reaction. You can keep pumping chemicals into your brain in an attempt to keep high arousal going, but sooner, rather than later, the system collapses into depression. This is known as the second law of libido or LL2. The first law of libido, by the way is: All drives regenerate so that recurrence is inevitable (LL1).

14.1.10 GIT-Brain Connection

If we think of the arousal system, SANDOH, as it functions in the body we can think of various complications as SANDOH is fed by blood vessels bringing materials from GIT. GIT and SANDOH form the principle stream of molecular information from the environment to our conscious experience. This molecular stream, as we have seen contains food products. Technically, these food products are heterogeneous populations of molecular species which titillate SANDOH in a variety of ways. There are many filters and buffers in the path from the GIT to SANDOH, but a surprising amount of the "wrong stuff" can get through. The first filter is the liver, also a chemical factory that transforms the molecules coming from GIT - 70% of incoming amino acids, for example, are removed and destroyed by the liver. Blood sugar and fat levels are regulated by the liver. The last filter before SANDOH is the Blood Brain Barrier (BBB), an imperfect defense. If the permeability of BBB is increased, major brain dysfunction can be expected. Immune-mediated diseases of the brain are among the most severe and disabling of human diseases - it is possible to imagine that these diseases occur if food allergens gain entrance to the brain through a defective BBB.

More routine problems of the "wrong stuff" reaching the brain produces typical arousal symptoms. Fatigue, sleepiness, mood and sleep disturbances are consistent symptoms of the food allergy complex. Many children become dopey or sleepy after eating. If there is no opportunity to sleep after the meal, they continue to function at a compromised level, making more mistakes in their work, and having more difficulty with interpersonal relationships. Children show distractability, irritability, restlessness, inattention, and failure to follow classroom lessons or failure to complete assignments.

Milk products, egg white, and cereal grains, especially wheat, seem to be the most consistent sedative-hypnotic-depressant foods. In children agitation, restelssness, and hyperactivity are associated with allergic symptoms (eg. flushing, congestion). All foods high in protein content may have this effect. The ideas that food should be selected to provide specific amino acids or specific protein-carbohydrate ratios does not work in practice because of the enormous potential for certain proteins to do harm before they are broken down to individual amino acids. Food molecules, especially intact proteins or pieces of protein probably interact with circulating immune cells which release chemical mediators. These mediators in turn influence brain function. Hyperarousal (irritability, agitation, hyperactivity, anxiety, fear) may accompany the circulating immune responses to ingested material (food allergy) and many adult patients report a restless, agitated state of mind or panic. Children act-out this state, but cannot describe or explain it. It is futile to ask a child "...why are you doing that?"

The emergency arousal state corresponds to the "fight and flight" sympathetic nervous system, built into animal brains for millions of years. Itching is a milder, but still disturbing hyperarousal. Skin itching is a symptom which focuses this hyperarousal. More generalized internal "itchiness" is also reported by adults. Children are unable to accurately described their feelings, but may refer to insects crawling on their skin, burning sensations, or itching. We observe their scratching, squirming, repeated movements (rocking, head-banging), bizarre behavior, agitated searches for relief, or restless, aimless, disorganized behavior.

A cruel paradox of sleepiness accompanied by restless dysphoria is often experienced at night while the evening's food and drink are being processed in the gastrointestinal tract and wrong materials trickle into the blood stream. Children sweat through the night, wet the bed, wake up frequently and wander into their parents' room (if permitted), or awaken with night terrors or memories of horrific nightmares. In the morning they are often hard to arouse, irritable, and disorganized.

Since the brain's arousal circuits determine our ability to attend to tasks, disturbances in the arousal system will manifest as attention deficits. The symptoms of difficulty in concentration, easy distractability, and memory deficit (most often failure to store recent memories) accompany other arousal dysfunction in both children and adults. Attention deficits in children are often cause "learning disability".

New 21st century psychotherapy is based on the concept that - whenever the buffers and filters between the GIT and SANDOH are breached, food and beverage input through the mouth should cease, to be replaced by a safer and more compatible input of an Elementary Nutrient Formula, custom-formulated to suit the needs of SANDOH. Only when food is replaced by nutrient formulas (ENFood) can we meaningfully regulate arousal and mood by changing the proportions of different amino acids, carbohydrates, and fatty acids. This is the domain of Molecular Programming. To fully restore mental health, input of toxins through the lungs should also cease, replaced by clean, filtered, humidified air. In a utopian world, information input would also be organized into a coherent, harmonious, stream of world events, which would gently persuade us not to be afraid of the universe.

14.2 Attention Deficit Hyperactivity Disorder

Learning disabilities (LD) may arise for hundreds of different reasons. The most prevalent form of LD afflicts children with normal intelligence and no specific handicaps. They have difficulty concentrating on tasks, are easily distracted, and cannot maintain an organized sequence of tasks. They fail to remember instructions and do not retain information well. Their failure in school gives them an enormous inferiority complex, which often becomes a bigger problem than the original LD. Their problems remain a puzzle to teachers, parents, psychologists, and physicians alike.

In psychiatric nomenclature, the diagnosis is "Attention Deficit Hyperactivity Disorder", ADHD. We can refer to attention deficit disorder (ADD) with or without hyperactivity. Thus we can have ADD or AD + Hyperactivity Disorder (ADHD). Hyperactivity can also occur without attention deficits, although this is difficult to appreciate in the classroom setting. Hyperactivity tends to now be called the "Hyperkinetic Syndrome". These are descriptive terms for restless, distractible children who have a knack for disrupting any environment that tries to enclose and control them. They have poor impulse control, often display abrupt mood swings, have inappropriate anger, and sometimes are violent. Their schoolwork suffers from inattention, disorganization, poor memory, and behavior disruptive of an otherwise orderly classroom. They have average or above-average intelligence. ADHD may improve as children age, but many children are permanently handicapped by a combination of poor achievement, low self-esteem, antisocial behavior, and persisting problems of disorganized PsyE. It is likely that juvenile deliquency and, later, criminal adaptations are often linked to the ADD-H-LD complex.

Several theories have been advanced to explain ADHD. The theory of "minimal brain damage or dysfunction" has had many advocates. The child is viewed as having a fixed disability, manifesting a structural problem of brain, acquired during prenatal development or at birth. Language disability or dyslexia has also been attributed to a fixed circuitry problem in the brain which impairs encoding and decoding of language symbols.

These brain-damage theories ignore the living, dynamic properties of the brain; they seem to view the brain as a simple appliance or computer which comes hardwired to behave in a certain way. But what about the daily input of molecular substances to the brain? Can improper food-body-brain interactions, sustained by habitual food choices, produce the patterns of dysfunction commonly observed? Can we fix the problem by molecualr re-programming? To imagine a dietary solution to these problems is to imagine a compassionate, safe, inexpensive redemption of countless youngsters. The potential beneficial impact on society is enormous. The Core Diet is a prototype of this desirable solution.

14.2.1 Feingold Theory

Several unsuccessful dietary theories have been put forward to explain behavioral and learning abnormalities, especially hyperactivity. Dr. Feingold blamed salicylates and food dyes for ADD-H.[67] Careful reviews of his low-salicylate diet showed that a minority of hyperactive children benefited from food dye and salicylate exclusion diets. A "panel of experts" concluded that the salicylate elimination diet should not be universally applied to hyperactive children, but that "dietary management" may be warranted in selected children.[68] Unfortunately, many commentators on the food-behavior connection have generalized extravagantly from this conclusion. I often hear that "diet has nothing to do with hyperactivity", a reckless interpolation of the Feingold diet review. The good news is that the Core Diet goes far beyond the Feingold diet in solving the hyperactivity problem. With proper management, comprehensive in intent and adapted to the needs of individual children, the Core Diet should be very successful in ameliorating behavioral disturbances and learning disabilities in children.

14.2.2 Sugar Theories

"Sugar" is universally blamed for hyperactivity, with no important substantiation of this idea. The observation that childrens' behavior deteriorates after eating sugar-containing foods, such as chocolate chip cookies, cake, slushies, pop, strawberry ice cream, or chocolate bars, is so universal that the phenomenon "must be valid"; the sugar-hyperactivity connection illustrates a mistake of attribution, blaming the results of the complex interaction of many food ingredients with the body on only one of the ingredients. When sugar (glucose and sucrose) alone is given to children, they tend to be sedated, with unchanged or even decreased physical activity.[69]

The phenomena of "sugar" reactivity are better explained by the whole-systems approach. It may be that sugars potentiate the brain-altering effects of other food ingredients and, therefore, appear to be responsible for hyperactivity. Sugar, accompanying amino acids in food, alters brain synthesis of neurotransmitters and may be one of the many food-body interactions which produces behavioral effects. High doses of sugar have other profound metabolic effects and induce an unstable eating patterns, characterized by cravings for sweet foods and compulsive eating.

To understand the effects of "sugar", one must consider the metabolic consequences of each individual sugar. In previous discussions, we have assigned different roles to glucose, fructose, galactose, and mannose. We have also appreciated that dissacharides influence gastrointestinal tract function. As well, we have appreciated that complex carbohydrates function very differently from their component sugars.

Another popular sugar hypothesis suggests that hypoglycemia (low blood sugar) is responsible for irritability, fatigue, depression, and learning difficulties. Again, this hypothesis has not been substantiated and is too simplistic to be an adequate explanation of diverse forms of dysfunction. High sugar intake is never desirable for children, nor adults. The move to artifical sweeteners is also not desirable. The Core Diet encourages moderation of total sugar intake, but does not attribute dysfunctional problems to sugar alone. The high protein diets prescribed for alleged "hypoglycemia" are definitely not desirable for children.

We must look beyond popular notions, blaming sugar for all these complex behavioral problems to find the real culprits which are more elusive, and more complex in nature. Milk may become public enemy number one!

14.2.3 Neuroactive Chemicals

Other food ingredients have been named as the culprits in children's behavioral problems. The aromatic substances and "amines" in fruits, for example, are neuroactive chemicals which produce behavioral changes when given alone. Banana oil acts in some children as a neuroactive drug and gives credence to the popular phrase "Going Bananas". Bananas also contain dopamine, an important neurotransmitter. Most ingested dopamine is probably metabolized in our blood by the enzyme MAO and does not cross the blood brain barrier. Often the disturbing "Agent X" in the bananas are removed by cooking. The interesting point is that fruits, vegetables, and spices have a variety of neuroactive chemicals which we know very little about. Nutmeg is known to contain hallucinogenic substances, and cinnamon often triggers hyperactivity and/or headaches. Several naturally occurring polyphenolic compounds have been studied for their effects on behavior. Gallic acid, for example, suppresses food intake in animals. In rat studies, obese rats were more sensitive to appetite suppression by gallic acid than their lean litter mates.[70]

Dr. R. Gardner [71] advanced the hypothesis that the whole range of aromatic compounds in the food supply are chemically active and also allergenic. There is little doubt about the biochemical activity of the "phenolic" compounds, but no reliable information on their allergenicity. Dr. Gardner's idea that someone could be "desensitized" against aromatic chemicals neither fits the immunological, nor biochemical models of food-body interactions.

I am not convinced that children can be helped by "desensitization drops" of any kind. Often desensitization drops are expensive placebos. Removing the offending food-chemicals from the diet is the only sensible approach.

14.2.4 Psychopharmacology & Hyperactivity

The most researched neurochemical approach to hyperactivity is based on a drug-neurotransmitter model of brain function. The brain utilizes specific neurotransmitters in specific subsystems which interact complexly to produce our mental existence and behavior. The neurotransmitter model recognizes the functional specifications of neurotransmitter systems. The system using dopamine, for example, emerges in the ancient core brain and serves our most basic functions. The arising dopamine circuits form part of SANDOH, discussed earlier in relation to PsyE. The dopamine system is involved in reward-seeking behavior, sexual behavior, control of movement, regulation of pituitary-hormone secretion, and memory functions. Dysfunction in dopamine circuits erodes our mental and functional existence at its very roots. The neurotransmitter model is greatly influenced by the study of drug effects on the brain. A model of schizophrenia postulates increased or unregulated dopamine circuits and drugs which block dopamine activity ameliorate the schizophrenic syndrome. An interesting neurochemical relationship between hyperactivity and schizophrenia has been postulated, where the two conditions seem to have opposite features.

Disorders of arousal and attention are disorders of PsyE and manifest some sort of dysfunction of SANDOH, which generates and regulates PsyE. The psychopharmacological model is an oversimplication, but allows us to think more specifically about the interactions of different systems within SANDOH. The hyperactivity syndrome, or ADD-H, may be attributed to dopamine deficiency. Dopamine synthesis slowly increases as children grow and may not reach full capacity until late teens. This is one of the built-in maturation lags which prevents some children from assuming adult-like behavior in their early life. Dopamine in young animals exerts a protective influence against hyperactivity.[72] Since schizophrenia is associated with increased dopaminergic activity and is improved by dopamine-blocking agents, there is a reciprocal relationship between psychosis and hyperactivity. A simple neurochemical relationship might look like:

increasing dopamine

HYPERKINETIC --------------->   SCHIZOPHRENIA

(decreased focal attention)   (increased focal attention)

SYNDROME   <--------------   STEREOTYPY

decreasing dopamine

Dopamine is made from the amino acid, tyrosine, which is partly made from another amino acid, phenylalanine. An early NP idea was to modify the amino acid profile of the diet to encourage dopamine synthesis by augmenting intake of phenylalanine and tyrosine and supplying extra cofactor, VM.B6 (pyridoxine). A more direct drug approach is to utilize molecules that stimulate dopamine circuits or act like dopamine in the brain (Dopamine agonists). The brain alchemists hope is that drugs at the right dose and time may be of benefit, if you feel comfortable with their use, and most parents do not. The experimental drug options are Pemoline, L-dopa, bromocriptine, amantadine, and lergotrile.

14.2.5 Drug Therapy for ADHD

The most common drugs of use and abuse which increase dopaminergic activity are ritalin and amphetamines. The drugs may decrease hyperactivity while they increase stereotypy. Ritalin has become the "drug of choice" for children with ADHD. Any child treated with ritalin is moved from the hyperactivity end of the spectrum toward a schizophrenia-like state. Ideally, one could find a convenient mid-range dose and achieve normal functioning, but in real-world terms the brain is too complex to allow simple drug manoeuvers to work well.

Ritalin therapy poses many risks, some obvious and others concealed. The most obvious ritalin effect is appetite supression and retarded growth. Some parents complain that their ritalin-treated child acts like a "zombie". They describe emotional blunting and detachment from family and friends, a mild schizophrenic attribute. Children on higher doses and chronic use may manifest paranoid features - withdrawal, anger, restless, suspicious behavior. People who abuse amphetamines (speed freaks and diet-pill-poppers) regularly develop a psychotic state with paranoid features. Ritalin may also produce disruption of movement control in a few unlucky children. Facial and head tics may appear, and, in the Tourette's syndrome, progress to peculiar grunting and respiratory tics, associated with compulsive behaviors, manifesting stereotypy. The Tourette's syndrome is a frightening possibility in children treated with ritalin over a long period. No drug which works on the dopamine system is free of long term toxicity on the motor system.

Studies on the effects of long term ritalin use show us the mixed results we would expect from a symptomatic drug therapy which does nothing to remove the underlying cause of the disorder. In all drug-related studies of ADHD, there is no consideration of dietary variables, nor any thought that the learning and behavior problems are just symptoms of a more pervasive illness. The reviewers of drug studies discover that ADHD continues through adolescence into adult experience. The names for the disorder change as patients age and accumulate social and interpersonal problems. Dr. Gabrielle Weiss, for example, concluded that:[73]

> "1. Most studies show that about half of the probands (subjects) have "outgrown" the syndrome. However, one to two thirds of the subjects continue to evidence symptoms of the syndrome...
>
> 2. Most studies indicate that hyperactives have lower self-esteem and rate themselves and are rated higher by others on various indicators of pathology...
>
> 3. In all studies, it is evident that for a significant minority, hyperactivity in childhood leads to adult antisocial personality disorders..."

Dr. Lily Hechtman reviewed the outcome of children treated with ritalin.[74] She stated:

> "Thus, stimulant treatment in childhood does not seem to secure a positive adolescent outcome for the hyperactive. However, studies that have combined stimulants with other

> multimodal interventions... do suggest more positive
> outcomes."

Unfortunately, no "multimodal" program reviewed by Dr. Hechtman included proper diet revision therapy, and the few that were reported have divergent methods with ambiguous results. In our experience, the Core Diet replaces drug therapy in children who have well-motivated parents. We propose a multimodal therapy which repairs the attention deficit disorder with effective, diet revision therapy; repairs academic deficits by appropriate remedial education; repairs lost self-esteem by family and child counselling; and maintains normal functioning by supporting the family effort to sustain proper diet, learning and social opportunities. A brief review of our concepts follows in the next section.

14.3 The Food Allergy Model of ADHD

We treat ADHD as a symptom of an endemic illness. The same pattern of disturbance occurs in children of affluent countries throughout the world. This is certainly not a local, individual problem of bad parenting, or poor teaching, or just bad children. The symptoms and signs of ADHD tells us that a child suffers biological disturbances secondary to more global problems in his/her food supply. The food supply problems are an aspect of a maladaptive biogical problem. School failure and disturbed behavior is a biological problem with severe social consequences.

My clinical studies gravitated to the food allergy model as I realized from them that hypoallergenic diets were much more successful than other diets, drug therapy, and vitamin-mineral supplementation in helping children recover. We have correlated physical illness patterns with learning disabilities and behavioral problems. A typical profile of the illness patterns included the symptom complexes associated with food allergy.

The school profile of children with delayed pattern food allergies, involves a typical set of learning and behavioral problems. Teachers observe inattention, fluctuating performance, restlessness, distractibility, or aggressive behaviors, or remark on the quiet, withdrawn, disinterested nature of the child. Often the child is criticized for laziness or attention-seeking, or the parents are blamed for undisciplined behavior. Psychological evaluation often reveals average to above-average intelligence with attention deficits. Some will appear clumsy, with handwriting which varies from day to day, often appearing awkward or tremulous. The more seriously afflicted children will fail to learn properly and will require assessment and remediation. If the behavioral aberrancies are marked, they may be referred to school psychologists or psychiatrists. Difficulties in learning language skills top the list of learning problems and the diagnosis of dyslexia is often made. The irritable, restless child is considered "hyperactive" and may be disruptive in the classroom.

These children display quick mood shifts, tearfulness, aggressive behavior, and may, on occasion, be antisocial and violent. The symptoms of depression and hyperactivity may co-exist, alternate, or appear separately. Disruptive behavior in the classroom may be associated with refusal to follow instructions, trouble with classmates, and aggressive, sometimes violent behavior in the school yard.

The failure-complex has life-long implications, as the child's personality forms around the dysfunctional patterns. With persisting illness and failure, low self esteem, social maladaptation, and antisocial behaviours develop and may be the presenting problems. Unpleasant, oppositional behavior in the younger child grows into deliquent patterns in early adolescence, and, later, antisocial or criminal behavior, if uncorrected.

All of these symptoms may remit surprisingly and dramatically when food selection is changed and drugs discontinued. The details of a successful food plan vary from individual to individual. The most globally successful diet revision in all these illnesses involves complete revision of the problematic diet. Selective "elimination diets" tend not to work. The proper technique of diet revision therapy is designed to solve simultaneous problems in the child's food supply. Consideration is given to minimizing exposure to food additives, to choosing nourishing, primary, low allergenic foods as dietary staples, and to assuring nutrient adequacy by careful monitoring of the child's food intake. Nutrient supplementation is necessary and is provided on the basis of computed nutrient intake Inventories.

14.3.1 Research Confirmation

An excellent study, published by Dr. Egger and his colleagues in 1985, definitively demonstrates a food allergy mechanism in symptomatic, hyperactive children. Their summary is noteworthy:[75]

"The hyperkinetic syndrome is a poorly defined but seriously handicapping behavior disorder, probably of multiple etiology. Various forms of treatment, especially behavior modification and stimulant medication, have been reported to be effective. It has also been suggested that food colorants and preservatives sometimes cause the hyperkinetic syndrome, presumably by evoking an idiosyncratic response to their pharmacologically active constituents. However, results of double-blind, controlled trials to test this hypothesis have largely been negative, though individual patients may respond consistently to particular substances. A role for food allergy has also been postulated, but this has not been tested by appropriate trials. During a double-blind, controlled trial that showed that any combination of foods could cause migraine in children, we noted that many of the responders had also been overactive and that their overactivity usually improved with food avoidance, in some instances with avoidance of foods other than those causing migraine. We have therefore treated overactive children with an oligoantigenic diet (one containing few varieties of foods); in those who responded, we identified provoking foods by reintroducing foods sequentially, then undertook a randomized, crossover, placebo-controlled trial of the effect of reintroduction of these foods on the development of overactivity and associated symptoms.

"The sequential reintroduction of foods enabled us to identify the foods that adversely affected a child's behavior. The hypothesis that combinations of any foods can alter behavior (based on allergy theory) has been supported in double-blind, controlled trials, not only in the hyperkinetic syndrome but also in migraine. By contrast, trials based on the idiosyncracy hypothesis (tyramine in migraine and salicylates, colorants, and preservatives in behavior disorders) have produced largely negative results. All the same, colorants (tartrazine) and preservatives (benzoates) were the commonest substances that provoked abnormal behavior in our patients, although no patient in this series reacted to them alone. The foods to which these patients also reacted were not chemically related to tartrazine or benzoates, which can be antigenic and, unlike salicylates, have no established pharmacological activity. Feingold recommended avoiding natural salicylates as well as drugs and food additives which contained them or chemically similar substances; such foods include peaches and cucumber, which were very low in our list of symptom-producing foods. The results of this study are not inconsistent with the largely negative results of double-blind controlled trials of the effect of preservatives and colorants in hyperactive children, since we found that no child reacted to preservatives and colorants alone. Moreover, in at least two of the previous trials, the placebo and excipient was chocolate, which caused symptoms in 59% of our patients.

"We prefer the hypothesis of allergy, but allergy and idiosyncrasy could co-exist and be interrelated in a complex manner. We have found that patients with migraine no longer responded to such non-specific stimuli as exercise, heat, or trauma to the head if they avoided the foods to which they responded adversely. Such an effect could be expected with foods that had pharmacological actions but there is no evidence of this and no evidence that aniline dyes or benzoate have any pharmacological effects. More research is needed to explain why these substances, also important in some other allergic diseases, such as angio-oedema and eczema, are so prominent in this syndrome. However, they are particularly readily avoidable, since they have no nutritional value, and our findings strengthen the case for excluding them where possible from factory-processed foods and drugs...

"Response to diet was poorer when patients came from families exposed to adverse psychosocial factors, but more than half the children exposed to one or more unfavourable situations did respond, so they should not necessarily be regarded as unsuitable for treatment if the family seems cooperative. The effect of adverse psychosocial circumstances on response may be due to the multifactorial nature of this syndrome or perhaps to better compliance in families with favourable psychosocial backgrounds. In the case of children from adverse psychosocial environments who responded to the diet, the disturbances within the family might have arisen from food allergy in other family members, since food allergy is familial.

"Being on an acceptable diet did seem to make a remarkable difference to the lives of many of these families. Many of the children, however, still have considerable behavior problems, and they and their families continue to require counselling and advice concerning management of the child's behavior. Nevertheless, of the 62 children who responded, 57 (92%) were continuing the diet when last seen, despite the effort and expense involved. The observation that some patients ceased to react to certain foods suggests that recovery from this form of food allergy can occur, as it may in others."

Many physicians have described diet revision treatment for childrens' problems. Dr. Egger remarks:[76]

"A role for food allergy in the hyperkinetic syndrome has been postulated since early this century."

Unfortunately, the Feingold diet proved to be a smoke-screen and received exaggerated attention. When the limited benefits of the Fiengold program were publicized, many thoughless writer's took it to mean that "all diet therapy was of little or no benefit".

14.3.2 A Study of Children on the Core Diet

Dr. Julianne Conry, an educational psychologist at the University of British Columbia, joined me in 1986 to study the pyschological and educational experiences of the children I was treating. Our first collaborative project was to measure and document behavior and learning performance changes in a group of my young patients undergoing food allergy management.

The Core Diet for Kids

Dr. Conry and I selected 50 children from a larger group of children, presenting for medical management of physical symptoms, suggestive of food allergic disease. These children had associated learning difficulties, often with behavior disturbances. Of the 50 computer-selected children, 45 children completed Stage 1 (medical evaluation and psychometric evaluation). Medical evaluation included a detailed history questionnaire, physical examination, laboratory tests, and a food-symptom journal, kept for at least two weeks by the parents. Psychometric evaluation was carried by Dr. Conry and a group of post-graduate students in educational psychology. The post-graduate researchers followed the children they had evaluated by telephone contact with the parents and performed an end-of-study assessment 3-4 months after diet revision was instituted. The study selection criteria were designed to identify children with both physical symptoms and school dysfunction. Scores derived from the parents responses to the medical questionnaire were used to identify children with:

1. Total symptom scores greater than 15 (each major symptom was rated on a 0-3 scale);

2. A school difficulty score of 5 or greater (5 categories of school performance - reading, writing, spelling, arithmetic, all work -were also scored with 0-3 ratings of degree of difficulty);

3. Attention deficit and/or hyperactivity - score of 2 or 3 out of 3.

The group of 30 children that completed the study had the following characteristics:

1. Age range 6 to 11: 8 girls; 22 boys.
2. Grade range 1 to 6
3. The learning difficulty score 6 to 15

Symptom scores reflected the degree of recurring or chronic illness; the total score for symptoms during the preceding 6 months ranging from 18-85, Average 43. Symptoms scores relative to different body systems were highest for the respiratory tract (Range 2-30; Average 15). The commonest symptom was nasal congestion, followed by cough and sore throats. We have called the common respiratory symptom complex "CURS" for Chronic Upper Respiratory Syndrome -this includes the ear, nose and throat symptoms, typical of delayed-pattern food allergy. The majority of children had symptoms from disturbances in more than one body system. Gastrointestinal disturbances were second to respiratory (Range 0-24;Average 10). More than half the children suffered significant episodes of pain - headache, abdominal pain, and leg pains were the most Common (Range 0 -17; Average 6). The medical problem lists of the 40 children are included in the summary -up to 4 major medical problems were recorded. The majority of these children had been significantly ill during the first 5 years of their lives, with respiratory symptoms (CURS, and bronchitis or asthma) leading the problem lists (Range 7-51; Average 27).

The children were also initially rated on a 0-3 scale for difficulties in reading, writing, spelling, arithmetic, and all work; the average score in all academic performance items was 2, with a range of 0-3.

Behavioral problem ratings included:

hyperactivity	– 18
disruptive behavior	– 15
attention deficit	– 30
difficulties with peers	– 18

14.3.3 Diet Revision Strategy

The Core Diet was the treatment plan for the children in this study. The Core Diet has changed somewhat since the study. Its present form has slower food introductions, and the introduction of soya protein has been delayed. To review: the Core Diet begins with a hypoallergenic clearing week with rice, selected vegetables, selected fruits, and poultry. The children were maintained on this diet until symptom remission occurred, and then foods were progressively added in a specified sequence. If symptoms returned, the offending foods were identified and were removed from the food list. The parents kept a detailed food-intake-symptom record everyday and it was monitored by the attending physician at intervals of 3-4 weeks. Problems were solved at the physician visits, with counselling provided to resolve conflicts, dissatisfactions, and compliance problems. Many parents needed detailed instructions about food selection, preparation, compliance incentives, and symptom interpretation. All the children took a prescribed multiple vitamin-mineral supplement and calcium carbonate (500 mg) to assure adequate intake of micronutrients.

Each child has a unique set of problems, and successful diet revision therapy is, therefore, individualized and adjusted according to ongoing observations. The medical objective is remission of all symptoms. The study objective was to evaluate the impact of Diet Revision Therapy on the child's performance at school and at home. Included in the medical evaluation of improvement was consideration of improved mood, thought clarity, and behavior at home; teacher reports of school performance were also reviewed, along with report cards.

Medical assessment at four months found 19 of the children with complete symptomatic remission, improved behavior at home, and improved school performance. Partial remission of symptoms (at least 80% reduction) was achieved in 9 children, with symptoms often attributable to "cheating" on the dietary regime. 5 of these children proved to be hypersensitive, and were prone to recurrent viral illness, which complicated their management. 2 children showed only intermittent improvement –in one case because of poor compliance, in the other because of hypersensitivity to food and environmental allergens.

14.3.4 Difficulties Studying Diet-Behavior Relationship

There are many difficulties in carrying out studies of this complexity. The easiest science is done with one variable in the privacy and comfort of a laboratory, surrounded by supportive colleagues. Real-world science deals with great complexity, great uncertainty and many interacting variables. Skeptics who do not know what is really going on in the real world sometimes demand "proof" from research activities. In medicine, "proof" is a rare commodity; but there is an unusual belief in the value of "double-blind controlled studies" - a method of research that drug use made popular. This methodology works when one variable is being considered. The most refractory skeptics demand "double-blind" studies of diet revision therapy before they will consider it (without suggesting how this could possibly happen). In my opinion, this is not appropriate "scientific" skepticism, but a form of dogmatic resistance that conceals the truth. The Core Diet stragegy does not lend itself to double-blind methods of study. Instead, it requires fully awake, responsible collaboration of physicians, parents, teachers, and psychologists. There is no placebo effect involved over the long term. Indeed there is a strong anti-placebo effect. Both parents and children struggle against great reluctance to continue the core diet and may deny improvement as an excuse for quitting. Parents have numerous opportunities to observe the recurrence of symptoms and behavior problems when the wrong foods are eaten. The effort to achieve meaningful change and problem-solve is similar to most meaningful exercises in human existence, requiring intelligence, patience, and perseverance to solve technical and/or social problems.

We have realized that our efforts to measure childrens' performance, however meaningful, are often not fully indicative of the improvements in children that are most valuable to us. A school principal, for example, referred to their "miracle child", a boy who improved so dramatically on the Core Diet that he moved from special education classes to coping well with regular classroom work. Our measurements missed the important improvements in family dynamics and missed the increased well-being of the improved children with better relationships with siblings and friends. Psychometric measurements can show improvements, but seem to miss some of the most important parameters of behavior and school performance. Our one-time samples were specially unreliable since we were trying to observe a dynamically changing performance state. If we measured a child on a "good day", achieved by strict compliance with the core diet we tended to get favorable measurements. If we measured a child on a "bad day", because of exceptions to the Core Diet we would get measurements of the dysfunctional state. Obviously researchers will have to understand the difference between spot sample measurements which may change radically with the child's biological status, and averaged performance measurements which show the net effect over time of complex interventions like diet revision therapy.

Maintaining normal functioning in a highly allergic child can be difficult. Often teachers need special training, and awareness of food and environmental problems. The following excerpt is from a letter to Barbara Keeting, a special and compassionate teacher, who understands the needs of sick children with allergic disease. The letter describes a hypersensitive 8 year old boy with dramatic food and inhalant allergies:

"This 0 year old suffers from allergic disease. I have worked with him for almost eight months now and have seen significant improvement in his condition; however, he remains unusually sensitive to both food and environmental allergens and seems to need very close and careful management. His mother is dedicated to this very exacting task and seems to do well indeed. He has an attention deficit disorder with episodes of hyperactivity. We have observed on many occasions that an allergic response will trigger hyperactivity, often associated with aggression and, sometimes, alarming rage responses. In his worst moments he is known to have refractory temper tantrums, lasting up to several hours. His emotional stability has greatly improved with careful dietary management. We have found that he is limited to a very small number of safe foods, mostly common vegetables. He seems to do best with frequent small feedings. He also does best when his environment is stable and unchanging.

I appreciated your telephone report on his progress. I agree with you completely that he needs a great deal of individual attention and a stable school environment. It would be in his best interests to keep him in the same classroom as much as possible and to avoid, at least for the time being, moving him from class to class or from teacher to teacher. He will do well with one-to-one teaching, in a quiet calm classroom with few distractions. When he is doing well, he displays remarkable insights and seems bright and intelligent, with an active imagination. I am pleased that you are able to supervise his food and that it is possible for him to bring proper meals, cooked at home, and to eat at regular intervals during the day. This form of personalized management seems to keep him most stable. We should have some concern for air quality. He will do best if stays in a familiar, clean, well-ventilated room.

If he has a food allergic reaction with typical signs like flushing, nose congestion, agitation, and confusion, there is no effective antidote - management of his agitation and angry responses simply requires protecting him from injuring himself or others and waiting for the reaction to subside. Antihistamines seem to offer little benefit, although a Seldane tablet is worth trying."

14.3.5 Review of Food-Behavior Interactions

These are the basic arguments in seeking a theory of food-body-brain interactions in children:

1. The effect of diet can only been understood as a multidimensional matrix involving many body systems. The net effect impinges on brain function, influencing perceptual, cognitive, and behavioral processes.

2. Food can be viewed as the input to a multidimensional body-brain matrix. Brain dysfunction is expressed as disordered thinking, feeling, behaving, and remembering. Within the complex of dysfunctional patterns, food allergy has emerged as a unifying concept of the origin of many dysfunctional patterns, its critical role evaluated by strategies of diet revision.

3. The food allergy model postulates that foods immunize us against a very large number of antigens - this vast and continuously changing immunity produces, by a variety a mechanisms, dysfunction and disease, including brain dysfunction.

4. The new models of food allergy postulate several overlapping problems, including the wrong entry of large molecules into the bloodstream, through the intestinal wall. This wrong-entry triggers immune responses and otherwise disorders metabolic and biochemical processing in target organs.

5. The food allergy illness patterns in children involve typical clusters of digestive, respiratory, skin, and behavioral disturbances.

6. The illness patterns occasionally involve inhalant allergies, defined in the usual way by skin and blood tests, but are not related to the inhalant allergies and operate independently of any mechanism that has been defined by simple allergy diagnostic techniques.

Appendix A
FOOD LIST

PHASE 1	**PHASE 2**	Dates
Basic Foods	**Vegetables**	**Fish Options**
Rice	Celery	Sole
Rice cakes	Cauliflower	Halibut
Rice cereal	Lettuce	Cod
Pears	Asparagus	Tuna fish
Carrots	Turnip	
Peas	Cucumber	**Meat Options**
Peaches	Spinach	
Yams	Onions	Beef
Sweet Potatoes	Brussels Sprouts	Lamb
Green Beans		
Broccoli	**Rice Flour Baking**	**PHASE 3**
Zucchini		
Squash	Rice bread	**Flavorings**
Chicken	Brown rice	
Turkey	Rice flour	Vanilla
Water	Baking soda	Ketsup
	Baking powder	Soy sauce
Oils	Sugar	Vinegar
	Honey	Dill
Safflower Oil	Milk-free margarine	Bay leaves
Sunflower Oil		Celery seed
Olive oil	**Fruit**	Marjoram
Linseed Oil		Ginger
	Applesauce	Mustard
Condiments	Watermelon	Carob
	Honeydew	Lemon/Lime
Pepper	Cantaloupe	
Salt	Plums	**Seeds**
Rosemary	Apples	
Thyme	Strawberries	Sesame seeds
Oregano	Raspberries	Tahini
Basil	Blueberries	Sunflower seeds
Parsley	Avocado	Pumpkin seeds

Soy Products

Soy Milk
Soy infant formula
Tofu
Tofu products
Tofu ice cream

Legumes

Peanuts
Yellow wax beans
Lentils
Lima beans
Pinto beans
Split peas
Kidney beans
Chickpeas
Snowpeas

PHASE 4

Vegetables

Bok Choy
Cabbage

Beets
Leeks
Chard
Bean sprouts
Potatoes
Tomatoes
Pumpkin
Radish
Parsnip
Kale
Kohlrabi
Corn

Fruit

Pineapple
Apricots
Cranberries
Currants
Nectarines
Blackberries
Cherries
Mango
Papaya
Orange

Prunes

Seafood

Trout
Salmon
Prawns
Lobster
Crab
Abalone
Shrimp

Grain Substitutes

Buckwheat
Millet
Tapioca
Cornstarch
Arrowroot
Soy flour

Flavorings

Mint
Garlic

Appendix B
SUCCESSFUL CHILDREN'S CORE DIETS

The following are examples of the types of foods consumed by children who are successful on the Core Diet. The food lists represent one day's intake.
EXAMPLE OF SUCCESSFUL CHILD'S CORE DIET - AGE 8

FOOD LIST

Food Name	Serving	Portion	Amount
CEREAL-CREAM OF RICE-COOK	1.000	CUP	244.0 GMS
APPLES-RAW-UNPEELED	1.000	ITEM	138.0 GMS
WATER	2.000	CUPS	474.0 GMS
RICE CAKE-REGULAR	2.000	ITEMS	18.6 GMS
JAMS/PRESERVES-REGULAR	2.000	TEASPOONS	13.3 GMS
PEARS-RAW-BARTLET-UNPEELED	1.000	ITEM	166.0 GMS
LETTUCE-ICEBERG-RAW-CHOP	0.500	CUP	27.5 GMS
CUCUMBER-RAW-SLICED	0.500	CUP	52.0 GMS
CHIVES-RAW-CHOPPED	1.000	TABLESPOON	3.0 GMS
SAL DRESS-VINEGAR/OIL-HOME	1.000	TABLESPOON	15.6 GMS
SQUASH-WINTER-BAKE-MASH	1.000	CUP	205.0 GMS
PEAR NECTAR-CAN	0.500	CUP	125.0 GMS
FISH-TUNA WHITE-CAN/WATER	3.000	OUNCES	85.0 GMS
PEAS/CARROTS-FROZ-BOIL	1.000	CUP	160.0 GMS
BEANS-SNAP-GREEN-RAW-BOIL	0.500	CUP	62.5 GMS
BROCCOLI-RAW-BOIL-DRAIN	0.500	CUP	77.5 GMS
CEREAL-RICE-PUFFED-PLAIN	1.000	CUP	14.0 GMS
FORM-ISOMIL-ROSS	0.250	CUP	60.0 GMS
WATER	1.000	CUP	237.0 GMS
WATER	0.250	CUP	59.3 GMS
SALT-TABLE SALT	0.125	TEASPOON	0.6 GMS
BEANS-SNAP-GREEN-RAW-BOIL	1.000	CUP	125.0 GMS
RICE-WHITE-PARBOIL-COOKED	1.330	CUPS	232.8 GMS
CALCIUM 500 MG	1.000	ITEM	1.0 GMS
NU-LIFE CHELA CAL-MAG	1.000	ITEM	1.0 GMS
SALT-TABLE SALT	0.250	TEASPOON	1.3 GMS
PEAS-GREEN-FROZ-BOIL-DRAIN	0.250	CUP	40.0 GMS
SODIUM FLUORIDE 1.21MG+1MG	2.000	ITEMS	2.0 GMS
CARROT-RAW-WHOLE-SCRAPED	1.000	ITEM	72.0 GMS
RASPBERRIES-RAW	0.250	CUP	30.8 GMS
NUBEAR CHILDREN'S	1.000	ITEM	1.0 GMS
YAMS-BOIL OR BAKE-DRAIN	0.500	CUP	68.0 GMS
RICE-WHITE-PARBOIL-COOKED	1.000	CUP	175.0 GMS
VEGETABLE OIL-SAFFLOWER	0.250	TEASPOON	1.1 GMS
VEGETABLE OIL-SAFFLOWER	0.250	TEASPOON	1.1 GMS
VEGETABLE OIL-SAFFLOWER	3.000	TEASPOONS	13.6 GMS

The Core Diet for Kids

NUTRIENT ANALYSIS

```
NUTRIENT      RDA Type:    CHILDREN-7 TO 10 YEARS              Amount

KCALORIES     ]==================                             1754 Kc
PROTEIN       ]===================================            56.02 Gm
CARBOHYDRATE  ]=====================                          321.8 Gm
FAT           ]=========                                      33.49 Gm
LINOLEIC FA   ]=========                                      16.65 Gm
SODIUM        ]=========================                      1346 Mg
POTASSIUM     ]=============================================  3747 Mg
MAGNESIUM     ]==========================================================  550.5 Mg
IRON          ]==================================================  21.50 Mg
ZINC          ]==================================================  25.01 Mg
VITAMIN A     ]==============================================  48179 IU
VITAMIN D     ]===============================                548.5 IU
VITAMIN C     ]=================================================  212.1 Mg
THIAMIN       ]=================================================  6.670 Mg
RIBOFLAVIN    ]=================================================  5.890 Mg
NIACIN        ]=================================================  39.45 Mg
VITAMIN B6    ]=================================================  7.843 Mg
FOLACIN       ]=========================================      466.0 Ug
VITAMIN B12   ]=================================================  10.18 Ug
PANTO- ACID   ]=================================================  21.20 Mg
CALCIUM       ]=========================================      1349 Mg
PHOSPHORUS    ]=====================                          698.8 Mg
TRYPTOPHAN    ]=================================================  809.2 Mg
THREONINE     ]=================================================  3067 Mg
ISOLEUCINE    ]=================================================  3305 Mg
LEUCINE       ]=================================================  5888 Mg
LYSINE        ]=================================================  4435 Mg
METHIONINE    ]=================================================  1576 Mg
CYSTINE       ]=================================================  870.0 Mg
PHENYL-ANINE  ]=================================================  3280 Mg
TYROSINE      ]=================================================  2758 Mg
VALINE        ]=================================================  4383 Mg
HISTIDINE     ]===========================================    1644 Mg
COPPER        ]================================               2.940 Mg
MANGANESE     ]==============================================  8.334 Mg
IODINE        ]============================                   134.8 Ug
FLUORIDE      ]==========================                     2197 Ug
MOLYBDENUM    ]==============================================  215.8 Ug
VITAMIN K     ]=================================================  858.2 Ug
SELENIUM      ]===========                                    0.097 Mg
BIOTIN        ]==============                                 72.82 Ug
CHLORIDE      ]=                                              32.00 Mg
CHROMIUM      ]========================                       0.203 Mg

     % RDA:  ^0      ^40     ^80      ^120     ^160    ^200

          3004 GM    1754 KC   H2O: 86%    $4.04

     PROTEIN: 12%    CARBOHYDRATE: 71%    FAT: 17%
```

EXAMPLE OF SUCCESSFUL CHILD'S CORE DIET - AGE 15

FOOD LIST

Food Name	Serving	Portion	Amount	
RICE-WHITE-PARBOIL-COOKED	1.000	CUP	175.0	GMS
PEACHES-CAN/WATER PACK	1.000	CUP	244.0	GMS
TURKEY-LIGHT-NO SKIN-ROAST	3.000	OUNCES	85.1	GMS
CELERY-PASCAL-RAW-STALK	1.500	OUNCES	42.5	GMS
CARROT-RAW-WHOLE-SCRAPED	1.500	OUNCES	42.5	GMS
WATER	1.000	CUP	237.0	GMS
SQUASH-WINTER-BAKE-MASH	1.000	CUP	205.0	GMS
CAULIFLOWER-FROZ-BOIL	1.000	CUP	180.0	GMS
CARROTS-BOIL-DRAIN-SLICED	0.250	CUP	39.0	GMS
BLUEBERRIES-RAW	0.500	CUP	72.5	GMS
APPLES-RAW-UNPEELED	1.000	ITEM	138.0	GMS
WATER	1.000	CUP	237.0	GMS
FISH-HALIBUT-BROILED-DRY	4.000	OUNCES	113.4	GMS
RICE-WHITE-PARBOIL-COOKED	1.000	CUP	175.0	GMS
CELERY-PASCAL-RAW-DICED	0.250	CUP	30.0	GMS
ONIONS-MATURE-BOIL-DRAIN	1.000	TABLESPOON	13.1	GMS
PEAS-GREEN-FROZ-BOIL-DRAIN	0.250	CUP	40.0	GMS
CARROTS-BOIL-DRAIN-SLICED	0.500	CUP	78.0	GMS
BROCCOLI-FROZ-BOIL-DRAIN	0.500	CUP	92.5	GMS
APPLE JUICE-CANNED/BOTTLED	0.500	CUP	124.0	GMS
BLUEBERRIES-RAW	1.000	CUP	145.0	GMS
PEAS-GREEN-FROZ-BOIL-DRAIN	0.500	CUP	80.0	GMS
YAMS-BOIL OR BAKE-DRAIN	0.500	CUP	68.0	GMS
RICE-WHITE-PARBOIL-COOKED	0.500	CUP	87.5	GMS
SALT-TABLE SALT	0.125	TEASPOON	0.6	GMS
BEANS-SNAP-GREEN-RAW-BOIL	0.500	CUP	62.5	GMS
SALT-TABLE SALT	0.125	TEASPOON	0.6	GMS
RICE CAKE-REGULAR	2.000	ITEMS	18.6	GMS
FISH-SHRIMP-MEAT-CAN	2.000	OUNCES	56.7	GMS
VEGETABLE OIL-OLIVE	1.000	TEASPOON	4.5	GMS
SPINACH-RAW-BOIL-DRAIN	0.500	CUP	90.0	GMS
SALT-TABLE SALT	0.125	TEASPOON	0.6	GMS
SALT-TABLE SALT	0.250	TEASPOON	1.3	GMS
SEEDS-SUNFLOWER-DRIED	0.250	CUP	36.0	GMS
CALCIUM 500 MG	1.000	ITEM	1.0	GMS
VITAMIN A 2500 IU	4.000	ITEMS	4.0	GMS
VITAMIN D 200 IU	2.000	ITEMS	2.0	GMS
ADDED PROTECTION III	3.000	GRAMS	3.0	GMS
SODIUM FLUORIDE 1.21MG+1MG	2.000	ITEMS	2.0	GMS
SPINACH-RAW-BOIL-DRAIN	0.750	CUP	135.0	GMS

-- References and Notes --

1. Brody J. Good Food Book. 1987; Bantam Edition
2. Brody J. Nutrition Book. 1987; Bantam revised edition
3. Deslauriers M. A Parent's perspective on Delayed Pattern Food Allergy. New Westminster, BC: Family Place (newsletter), July 1989.
4. Selye H. The stress of life. New York: McGraw-Hill, 1956.
5. Good RA, Fernandes G, West A. Nutrition and immunity. Washington, DC: Nutrition Found., 1984.
6. Buscinco L et al. Epidemiology, incidence and clinical aspects of food allergy. Annals Of Allergy 1984;53:615-622.
7. Buscinco L et al. The spectrum of food allergy in infancy and childhood. Annals of Allergy 1986;57:213-218.
8. Hill D. Clinical recognition of the child with food allergy. Annals of Allergy 1987;59:141-145.
9. Brostroff J, Challacombe SJ. Food allergy and intolerance. England: Bailliere Tindall, 1987.
10. Hughes EC. Use of a chemically defined diet in the diagnosis of food sensitivities and the determination of offending foods. Ann Allergy 1978;40:393-398.
11. Dockhorn RJ, Smith TC. Use of a chemically defined hypoallergenic diet (Vivonex) in the management of patients with suspected food allergy/intolerance. Ann Allergy 1981;47(4):264-269.
12. Villavences JW, Heiner DC. Experience with an elemental diet (Vivonex). Ann Allergy 1985;55:783-789.
13. ENFood is a registered trade mark of EnVironMed Research Inc. 3661 W. 4th Ave. Vancouver, BC V6R 1P2 (604) 731-9168.
14. Quest Vitamin Supplies Ltd. 1781 W. 75th Ave. Vancouver, BC Canada. V6P 6P2 (604) 261-0611.
15. Whitehead RG. Nutritional aspects of human lactation. Lancet Jan. 22 1983;167-169.
16. Gerrard JW, Perelmutter L. IgE mediated allergy to peanut, cow's milk, and egg in children with special reference to maternal diet. 1986;56:351-354.
17. Owen LA. Feeding guide, nutritional guide for the maturing infant. Bloomfield, NJ: Mead Johnson and Health Learning Systems, November 1979.
18. Zee P. JAMA 1985;253:3269-3272.
19. Dietz WH and Gortmaker SL. Pediatrics 1985;75:807-812.
20. Issenman RM et al. CMAJ 1985;132:781-4.
21. Breskin MW. Journ Am Dietetic Assn 1985;85:49-56.
22. AminoAcids: Essential and Non-essential. Jackson A.A. Lancet. May 7 1983;1034-1037.
23. Horrobin DF. Clinical uses of fatty acids. Eden Press Inc, 1982.
24. Hegsted DM. Jour Nutrition 1986;116:478-481.
25. Food and Nutrition Board, National Research Council; Recommended Dietary Allowances, 9th edition. Washington DC: National Academy of Sciences, 1980.
26. Davis DR. Nutritional needs and biochemical diversity in medical applications of clinical nutrition New Caanan Conn: Keats Publ, 1983;41-63.
27. Gilchrist A. Foodborne disease & food safety. Monroe, WI: Am Med Ass'n, 1981.

28. Freydberg N, Gortner WA. The food additives book. New York: Bantam Books, 1982.

29. Furia TE. Food additives. Florida: CRC Press, 1973:1, 1980:11.

30. Tannenbaum SR. N-nitroso compounds: a perspective on human exposure. Lancet 1983;629-632.

31. Laseter JL. Chlorinated hydrocarbon pesticides in environmentally sensitive patients. Clin. Ecol. 1983;I,II:3-12.

32. McGuire R. Dioxin shock hits home. Medical Post November 1986;22(39):1,12.

33. Anon. Bad apples. Consumer Reports May 1989; 288-292.

34. Rea WJ et al. Pesticides & brain-function changes in a controlled environment. Clin Ecol. 1984;II(3):145-150.

35. Annest JL ot al. Chronological trends in blood lead levels between 1976 and 1980. NEJM 308(23):1373-1377.

36. Soderman JV. Identified carcinogens and noncarcinogens: carcinogenicity-mutagenicity database. CRC Press, Chemical Class File, 1981:1, Target Organ File 1981:2 Cat #3200BF.

37. Stich HF. Carcinogens and mutagens in the environment. CRC Press, Food Products, 1982:1 Cat #5882BF.

38. Reddy BS, Cohen LH. Diet, nutrition, and cancer: a critical evaluation. Florida: CRC Press, 1985:1 Cat #6332BF, 1986:2 Cat #6333BF.

39. Coca AF, Cooke RA. On the classification of the phenomena of hypersensitiveness. J Immunol 1925;10:445.

40. Cantani A, Buscinco E, Beninicori N. A three year controlled study in children with pollinosis treated with immunotherapy. Annals of Allergy 1984;53:79-84.

41. Gardner MLG. Evidence for, and implications of, passage of intact peptides across the intestinal mucosa. Biochem. Soc Trans 1983;11:813

42. Reinhardt MC. Macromolecular absorption of food antigens in health and disease. Ann Allergy 1984;53:597-601.

43. McNelsh AS. Enzymatic maturation of the gastrointestinal tract and its relevance to food allergy and intolerance in infancy. Ann Allergy 1984;53:643.

44. Bienstock J. Mucosal barrier functions. Nutr Reviews 1984;42(3)105-116.

45. Coombs RRA and McLaughlan P. Ann Allergy 1984;53:592.

46. Gerrard JW et al. Cow's milk allergy: prevelance and manifestations in an unselected series of newborns. Acta Pediat Scand Suppl 1973;234:2.

47. Hill DJ. Cow's milk allergy in infants: some clinical and immunologic al features. Annals of Allergy 1986;57:225-228.

48. Businco L et al. The spectrum of food allergy in infancy and childhood. Annals of Allergy 1986;57:213-218.

49. Wilson NW, Hamburger RN. Allergy to Cow's Milk in the first year of life and its prevention. Annals of Allergy 1908;61:323-328

50. Deamer WD, Gerrard JW, Speor F. Cow's milk allergy: a critical review. J Fam Prac 1979;9:223.

51. Ross Laboratories. Cow milk allergy. (Booklet). Montreal: April 1980; associated bibliography.

52. Novak M et al. The effect of a L-carnitine supplemented soyabean fromula on the plasma lipids of infants. Acta Chirurgica Scand Suppl 1983;517:149-155.

53. Unsworth DJ et al. IgA anti-gliadin antibodies in celiac disease. Clin Exp Immunol 1981;46:286-93.

54. Keiffer M et al. Wheat gliadin fractions and other cereal antigens reactive with antibodies in the sera of of celiac patients. Clin Exp Immunol 1982;50:651-60.

55. Bell L, Hoffer M. Recommendations for foods of questionable acceptance for patients with celiac disease. J Can Dietetic Ass'n 1981;42(2):143-158.

56. Physicians Cyto Laboratories of Florida Inc 1986.

57. Learey HL, Halsey JF. An assay to measure antigen-specific immune complexes in food-allergy patients. Jour Allergy Clin Immun 1984;74:(2)190-195.
58. Crook WG. The yeast connection. 1984.
59. Vaginitis blamed on prostaglandin production. Med Post October 29, 1985:34.
60. Morley JE, Levine AS et al. Effect of exorphins on gastrointestinal function, hormonal release, and appetite. Gastroenterology. 1983;84(6):1517-23.
61. Loukas S, Varoucha D, Zioudrou C et al. Opioid activities and structures of casein-derived exorphins. Biochemistry 1983;22:4567-4573.
62. Bobner, RF. Marchionda LM, Benz CR. et al. Behavioral Disorders A Nutrition Checklist. Academic Therapy. 1982 17:4 457-484.
63. Bates C. Personal communication. 1985. See also Bates C. Essential fatty acids & immunity in mental health. Tacoma WA: Life Sciences Press, 1987.
64. Aas K. General Discussion. Nutr Rev 1984;42(3):119.
65. Wurtman JJ. Managing your mind through food. New York: Harper & Row, 1988.
66. Weiss JM, Simson PG. Neurochemical basis of stress induced depression. Psychopharm Bul. 1985:21;447-457.
67. Feingold BF. Hyperkinesis and learning disabilities linked to artificial food flavours and colours. Am Jour Nursing 1979;75:797.
68. National Institute of Health, Concensus, Development Conference Draft Statement. Defined diets and childhood hyperactivity. Washington DC: NIH, 1982.
69. Behar D et al. Sugar challenge testing with children considered behaviorally "sugar reactive". Nutrition and Behavior 1984;1:277-288.
70. Glick Z, Oku J, Bray G. Effects of polyphenols on food intake and body weight of lean and obese rats. Nutrition and Behavior 1982;1:75-78.
71. Gardner R. Aromatic heterocyclic compounds as principal inciters of allergic responses. Soc Clin Ecol:14th Seminar Ed.
72. Margolin D. Hyperkinetic child syndrome and brain monoamines: pharmacology and therapeutic implications. Journ. of Clin. Psych. 1978;12-130.
73. Weiss G. Followup studies on outcome of hyperactive children. Psychopharm Bul. 1985;21(2):169-177.
74. Hechtman L. Adolescent outcome of hyperactive children treated with stimulants in childhood: a review. Psychopharm Bul. 1985;21(2):178-191.
75. Egger AU et al. Controlled trial of oligoantigenic treatment in the hyperkinetic syndrome. Lancet 1985;8428(I):540-545.
76. Egger J. The Hyperkinetic Syndrome. In Food Allergy. Brostroff and Challacombe eds. 1987; 674-687. Bailliere Tindell

Index

Mail Order Form

For Additional Books: Core Diet for Kids

# COPIES	Cover price	DISCOUNT	Our price
5	$79.75	10%	$71.77
ˑ5		20%	

We pay postage if order is PREPAID.

I would like to order

_____ COPIES   of the Core Diet For Kids

PAYMENT:

_____ Cheque/Money Order Enclosed

_____ Bill my Visa # _____

Signature _____ Bank _____

Expiry Date _____

Send to:

EnVironMed Research Inc.
#1-3661 West 4th Ave.
Vancouver, B.C.
V6R 1P2

Mail Order Form

For Nutritional Analysis and/or CORE DIET COOKING

I would like to order the following:

_____ Nutritional Analysis form - PREPAID $16.00 (Cdn funds)

_____ Core Diet Cooking - PREPAID $14.95 (Cdn funds) plus
postage and handling.

_____ Nutritional Analysis Form plus Core Diet Cooking -
PREPAID $24.95 (Cdn funds) plus postage and handling.

PAYMENT

_____ Cheque/Money Order Enclosed

_____ Bill my Visa # _____

Signature_____ Bank _____

Expiry Date _____

Send to:
NUTRIDATA
#1-3661 West Fourth Avenue
Vancouver, B.C.
CANADA
V6R 1P2